The
Raw Truth
RECHARGE

The Essential Guide To
Faith, Family, Food, Fitness

The
Raw Truth
RECHARGE

7 Truths For Total
Health and Fitness

ROBBIE RAUGH, RN

Board Certified
Integrative Heath and Nutrition Practitioner

Bridge-Logos, Inc.
Newberry, FL 32669

The Raw Truth Recharge
7 Truths For Total Health and Fitness
by Robbie Raugh, RN

Library of Congress Catalog Card Number: 2019932105
International Standard Book Number: 978-1-61036-403-4

Unless otherwise indicated, all Scripture quotations are taken from the Holy Bible, New Living Translation, copyright © 1996, 2004, 2015 by Tyndale House Foundation. Used by permission of Tyndale House Publishers, Inc., Carol Stream, Illinois 60188. All rights reserved.

Scripture quotations designated NIV are The Holy Bible, New International Version®, NIV® Copyright © 1973, 1978, 1984, 2011 by Biblica, Inc.® Used by permission. All rights reserved worldwide.

Scripture quotations designated TLB are from The Living Bible, © 1971 by Tyndale House Foundation. Used by permission of Tyndale House Publishers Inc., Carol Stream, Illinois 60188. All rights reserved.

Scripture quotations designated NKJV are from the New King James Version, © 1982 by Thomas Nelson. Used by permission. All rights reserved.

Scripture quotations designated The Message are from The Message. Copyright © 1993, 1994, 1995, 1996, 2000, 2001, 2002. Used by permission of NavPress Publishing Group.
Scripture quotations designated KJV are from the King James Version.

Robbie's front cover photo by Raquelle Raugh
Robbie's back cover bio photo by Raquelle Raugh
Robbie and Mom's photo by Sarah Bridgeman
Robbie's Family Photo by Boryana Georgiev
Interior Illustrations by Elaine Kessel

Disclaimer
The content of this book is for general instruction only. Each person's physical, emotional, and spiritual condition is unique. The instruction in this book is not intended to replace or interrupt the reader's relationship with a physician or other professional. Please consult your doctor for matters pertaining to your specific health and diet. Check with your doctor before starting any exercise or healthy eating protocol.

VP 01 06/2019

"You will spend the time and the money either way: you will either spend the time and the money treating disease; or you will spend the time and the money preventing disease by exercising and eating right.
Which is better for you?"
—Robbie Raugh, RN

"The doctor of the future will give no medication but will interest his patients in the care of the human frame, diet, and in the cause and prevention of disease."
—Thomas Edison

"Let food be thy medicine, and medicine be thy food."
—Hippocrates,
the father of modern medicine

"You can't fix your health until you fix your diet."
—Robbie Raugh, RN

"What you put on the end of your fork can either prevent disease or cause disease. Nothing changes if nothing changes, and yesterday you said tomorrow".
—Robbie Raugh, RN

DEDICATIONS

To my amazing husband Jeff, who has stood by me as I try to balance life, while following my dreams and calling.
Thank you and I love you.

To my beautiful daughter Shanelle who inspires me with her incredible work ethic and passion to care for others. I love you.

To my beautiful daughter Raquelle, who inspires me with her incredible talent and passion to glorify and honor God. I love you.

To my Dear Sister Susan, brother in-law Bill, my nieces Jessica, Amanda, nephew Ryan and their families I love you all.

To my nephews, Chris, Mike, Aaron and Keith Wallak, who have been like my own kids, and to my brother-in-law George. Thank you for teaching me strength and perseverance through life's trials and tribulations. I love you all.

My sisters-in-law Barbie, Suzette and Rosie, my brother-in-law Wally, their families, and Mom and Dad Raugh. I love you all.

To my Lord and Savior

Who died so that I could live. Thank you for the breath in my lungs and the beat of my heart. Thank you for rescuing me from sinking sand and putting me on solid rock. I pray that you speak through me with this book, and decrease me, increase You. My allegiance is forever to you, Lord Jesus. None of this would be possible, nor would it matter, without you.

IN MEMORY OF

My dear mom, Terry Palmisano, who instilled the belief in me that I could do anything I set my mind to, because she and God both loved me.

My dear dad, Robert Palmisano, who inspired me to live out my dreams with the gifts God gave me, as he himself did as an accomplished artist.

My dear sister, Arlene Wallak, who fought the most courageous battle with cancer I had ever witnessed. Her fight to live inspired me to fight for a cure and dive into the research of food as medicine, and become a disciple to save lives. Because of Arlene, I believe this is now my calling.

~Absent with the body means present with the Lord~

Even though I walk through the valley of the shadow of death, I will fear no evil, for you are with me; your rod and your staff they comfort me. (Psalm 23:4)

FOREWORD

ROBBIE RAUGH IS a dedicated motivator. She is an internationally known fitness trainer, a registered nurse, and a wellness expert. She has her own radio show in Western New York, and most of all, she is the epitome of the "practice what you preach" mentality. Robbie Raugh is all that and more, and she carries that passion and compassion into the writing of this book.

When I was asked to write the foreword for this book, I was not only truly honored, but excited to be even a small part of the achievements of the talented, multitasking, and formidable Robbie Raugh. I have known Robbie for more than two decades, and she has never wavered from her focus, putting the needs of her followers first and foremost.

"If I had to summarize my life and career in a few words, I would have to call myself a dedicated motivator," says Robbie. "Whether I am doing fitness training, one-on-one nutritional counseling, or on my weekly talk show, I am always trying to help others reach their ultimate best."

That may be the understatement of the century.

Robbie Raugh dedicates her life to the field of health and wellness. Starting out as a registered nurse, helping others, she transitioned to a thirty-year stint with Bally Total Fitness, reaching the ranks of National GE Director of 300+ clubs in two countries, overseeing more than 5,000 fitness instructors. As if that wasn't enough to fill her days, she embarked on a track to learn and teach nutrition and weight management, running several classes per week while working on a new venture for the Buffalo Athletic Club (BAC).

In addition to all of the above, Robbie appears regularly as the health and fitness expert on ABC-TV's AM Buffalo and hosts her own radio show on faith, family, food and fitness, The Raw Truth, on WDCX 99.5 FM, heard in the USA and Canada. She is also the featured instructor of four Raw Energy Fitness exercise videos and The Kinetic Workout Live exercise video, which has sold in 32 countries.

As a national fitness expert, she has presented at national conferences and conventions including the IDEA Health and Fitness Association and the Kingdom Bound International Christian Conference. She has been featured nationally on ESPN as having the largest regularly held class in

North America and her expertise has led to her being interviewed on TV and radio in the USA and Canada. Robbie has been featured in *Oxygen* and *Fitness* magazines.

After having lost her father, mother, and sister, Robbie began to recognize the link between diet, exercise, and lifestyle in preventing and reversing disease, and she now considers her work her "calling."

Robbie is equally dedicated to her husband and two daughters. When asked how she does all of this, she comments, "Well, I guess I just found a way to fit 25 hours in a day. I am blessed that God gave me the energy and drive to share my amazing life with others, helping them to achieve their optimum best through health and wellness."

This book, *The Raw Truth Recharge: 7 Truths for Total Health and Fitness*, is more than an exclamation point on her storied career. It is another chapter in her continued quest to rejuvenate the mind, body and soul of her followers. It captures Robbie's sense of focus on those things that create balance in our lives and make us better individuals to ourselves, our families, and our communities.

Robbie is truly a dedicated motivator through her actions as well as her words. Her enthusiasm toward motivating is contagious, and I hope you 'catch' her passion. As you read through this book, you will be treating yourself to an amazing perspective on creating total balance.

Dr. Samuel Shatkin, Jr.
www.drshatkin.com

ENDORSEMENTS

It would be near impossible in a few sentences, to describe the impact that Robbie Raugh has had on our lives and health. Yes, she is certified, qualified, and amazingly talented. But more than that, she sincerely cares about people, and wants them to prosper in every way. We would not be where we are today, without Robbie's love and guidance. This book will, without a doubt, transform your life.

—**Jill Kelly**
Wife of Jim Kelly
NY Times Best Selling Author, Speaker

—**Erin Kelly**
Daughter of Jim and Jill Kelly
Author, Speaker

The Raw Truth Recharge was written by a graduate of the Institute for Integrative Nutrition. If you are looking for a book to significantly improve the quality of your life, your health, and your vitality, I highly recommend you read this book and be in touch with Robbie Raugh, RN so your life can be the best life possible.

—**Joshua Rosenthal**
MScEd, Founder/Director, Institute for Integrative Nutrition

I have had the luck and pleasure of knowing Robbie for many years. Robbie Raugh is a consummate fitness professional. She has a deep understanding and many years of experience in the fitness and wellness industry. She has excelled in everything she has done, and once again, she brings her expertise and knowledge to this amazing and helpful book. I highly recommend this book; it is a great addition to any health, wellness and fitness library.

—**Carol Scott**
CEO – ECA World Fitness Alliance

This book is a must-read for anyone wanting to be healthy and fit! When I first met Robbie in my clinic in 2014, I knew there was something special about her. She's a strong Christian businesswoman who can improve the health of her clients better than many physicians can, despite their years of medical training. After hearing the success stories of multiple Raw Truth alumni, I knew Robbie was the individual I wanted to help me and my partners introduce healthy eating and living to our practice. We've had an amazing response from our patient population.

Since I'm the kind of guy who likes to test-drive any new service we introduce, I decided to join my partners and experience The Raw Truth Recharge for myself. I've been healthy my whole life, but a few years ago I had lab work done that showed some elevated liver enzymes. Despite my best efforts, I couldn't lower the numbers. I even had additional workups performed and a consultation with a specialist that left me with no definitive answers.

Four weeks after following Robbie's methods to remove harmful toxins from my body and eat a more natural and balanced diet, I had lab work done for my yearly physical. Miraculously, all my labs came back normal! What a powerful impression this made on me. Robbie's methods really work, and they can change your health and your life forever! The Raw Truth Recharge has my highest endorsement. You need to try it for yourself.

—**Dr. Michael Cicchetti, MD**
Partner, Buffalo Spine and Sports Medicine, PLLC

Robbie Raugh is passionate about life and faith. She is a leader, teaching us to have a healthier, Godly approach to food and fitness. This book will give you the tools to begin a journey to personal health and wellness.

Your health will be changed if you apply the principles she outlines in this book. Her never-ending energy and love for God shine through in everything she teaches. You will be blessed.

—**Donna Russo**
President Kingdom Bound Ministries

Endorsements

I have known Robbie for about five years and can testify to her passion for her Lord, family, and for people that they would experience the love of Christ and that they would experience health and balance. She was the first to give me some direction in terms of losing weight and equally important making wise choices in the things you eat. I believe that you will find her book to be of immense benefit to your physical health.

—Pastor Dave Drake
The Chapel at Crosspoint - Getzville NY

Robbie Raugh is truly a passionate fitness guru who loves to share her boundless knowledge with others to help them lead a more fit and healthy active life. Thousands have benefited from her experience and wisdom!

—Geoff Bagshaw
International Fitness Presenter
Group Fitness Manager at Equinox in NYC

In this book, Robbie will give you all the secrets to help transform your body, life and health, as she as done for so many of us. You will be blessed.

—Keri Cardinale
Talk Show Host "The Keri and Robbie Show" WDCX Radio

When I think of Robbie Raugh, I envision boundless energy that is matched only by her love of God, her family and her friends. Selfless and true, Robbie embodies a spirit of altruism that is unmatched by anyone else I've known. With her charisma, intelligence and compassion, Robbie can inspire in the gym, in the kitchen, in media settings or in the classroom. She has had an immeasurably positive influence on my life and my husband's and for that I am forever grateful. Robbie's expertise in this book will help educate and motivate all who read it.

—Brenda Alesii
Talk Show Host "A Slice of Life" ESPN radio

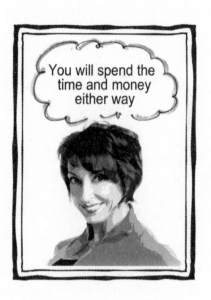

TESTIMONIALS

What Others Have Said About The Raw Truth Recharge

Robbie's passion for a healthy mind, body, and spirit are contagious! I've followed Robbie since the 1980s and have received a continuous education on fitness and healthy eating during her classes, through her 12-week healthy eating program, and online from her blog, website, and newsletters. Not even in medical school did I learn this level of science in nutrition and disease prevention that I can now share with patients and friends. I learned Nutrition at the Molecular level, not how to apply Nutrition to prevent and reverse disease. Thank you, Robbie, for keeping me current in this life changing and lifesaving discipline!

—**Dr. Terri Caligari**

I have faithfully attended Robbie's fitness classes for the past 19 years. She is truly an inspirational teacher who leads by example. I am impressed that her fitness program embraces three key fitness components. Cardio, resistance training and flexibility. I personally and professionally agree with her emphasis on commitment and consistency. With Robbie's expert instruction, I have achieved my goals of being fit, strong and reducing my stress level.

I selected my specialty of Pediatrics because it offers a unique opportunity to practice preventive medicine and care well for all my patients. Robbie has the same mission with her teachings. She offers classes on diet and lifestyle education, which focus on making daily healthy lifestyle choices. In turn she helps people prevent disease and improve their present and future health.

—**Dr. Lisa Reichert**

From above, down, inside and out, the power that made the body heals the body. Robbie Raugh truly exemplifies this paradigm. We incorporate The Raw Truth Recharge in helping our patients stay healthy, and feel great.

—**Dr. Matt Misiak**
Misiak Chiropractic

Table of Contents

INTRODUCTION

T HIS BOOK WOULD never be possible without God, nor would it even matter. From the breath in my lungs, to the beat of my heart, to the ability to type these words, I owe it all to Jesus.

My hope and prayer is that God gives me the words to educate, motivate, and inspire you in one way or another to live that abundant life that He desires for us in every arena of our life.

This book has seven truths. Why seven? Well, seven is the number of completeness and perfection, both physical and spiritual. It derives much of its meaning from being tied directly to God's creation of all things.

The number 7 is the foundation of God's Word.
First of all, God created the heavens and earth in six days and on the *seventh* day He rested. Then, Jesus performed *seven* miracles on God's holy Sabbath Day:

1. Cast an unclean spirit out of a man (Mark 1:21-28 and Luke 4:31-37)
2. Healed Peter's mother-in-law, who had a fever (Matthew 8:14-15, Mark 1:29-31 and Luke 4:38-39)
3. Healed a man's hand (Matthew 12:9-13, Mark 3:1-6 and Luke 6:6-11)
4. Healed a lame man by the pool of Bethesda (John 5:1-18)
5. Healed a crippled woman (Luke 13:10-17)
6. Healed a man with swollen limbs (Luke 14:1-6)
7. Healed a man born blind (John 9:1-7,14)

In Matthew 13, Jesus is quoted as giving seven parables:

1. Parable of the Four Soils
2. Parable of the Weeds
3. Parable of the Mustard Seed
4. Parable of the Yeast
5. Parable of the Hidden Treasure

6. Parable of the Pearl Merchant
7. Parable of the Fishing Net

Throughout the Bible, you will find references to the number seven:

- "Take with you seven of every kind" (Genesis 7:2)
- "March around the city seven times" (Joshua 6:4)
- "Seven that are detestable to Him" (Proverbs 6:16)
- "Comes, there will be seven sevens" (Deuteronomy 9:25)
- "Not seven times but seventy seven times" (Matthew 18:22)
- "To the seven churches in the Province of Asia" (Revelation 1:4)
- "Open the first of the seven seals" (Revelation 6:1)

And God has inspired me to share seven important truths with you, to hopefully help you to live the abundant life that God desires for all of us! God does not want us walking around sick and thick and tired—this I know! But it's much more than just physical health; it is truly mind-body-soul-spirit, all integrated.

It doesn't matter how much you eat right and exercise—if you don't pay attention to the truths I'm about to teach you, your health physically, mentally, emotionally, and spiritually will be starving. So if you are "in," let the transformation begin!

In order to write about life, first you must live it!
—Ernest Hemingway

To love what you do and feel that it matters.
How can anything be more fun?
—Robbie Raugh

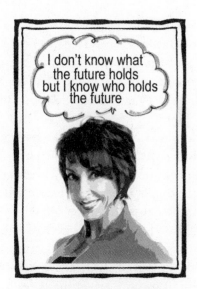

TRUTH ONE

Faith – Believe

Spiritual Fitness

Now faith is being sure of what we hope for and certain of what we do not see. (Hebrews 11:1)

THE TRUTH IS, without faith it is impossible to really do anything in life. You have to believe in what you are doing or what you want to do. Without faith, it's also impossible to please God, because anyone who comes to Him must believe that He exists, and that He rewards those who earnestly seek Him. I don't know what the future holds for you, but I do know WHO holds the future! It's God. The One who created the universe and everything in it including us, loves you and me. And actually, we were made by Him, and for Him, and until we understand that, nothing else will ever make sense.

Do you have your doubts that God even exists? I did, many times. We will talk about that, and why it's important to have faith, and how and why to believe.

1

There were times when I wondered where God was in my life. I believed He existed, but where was He when I needed Him? He wasn't there in the midst of my pain, or so I thought. As I grew older, and life became more complicated, I had more responsibility, and life was getting tough. I was so frustrated at times. So lost. I never blamed God; I just didn't know if He was really there.

But as I look back, God's hands were all over my life, even then. And although there were times that I drifted from Him, He never gave up on me. I can clearly recall countless times in my life that I cried out for Jesus, and although my faith was like the wind back then, He showed me His sovereignty and faithfulness time and time again.

His Word tells us that if we draw a line to Him, He will draw a line to us. That He will never leave or forsake us, and that when we live for Him, He will give us the desires of our heart. When I finally turned my life completely over to God, it was only then that I really saw the God I know today, and His sovereignty over my life.

Throughout the years, as my faith became stronger, God gave me the desires of my heart, and it wasn't a coincidence. I would even test Him saying, "God, if you are there, make this or that happen and show me a sign." How dare I put God to a test, but He always revealed Himself to me. Many prayers were answered, and I began to see His work in my life time and time again.

God will not make all your dreams come true just because you ask Him. You may be praying for something, and God gives you the opposite of your prayers. When this happens to believers, many nonbelievers ask "where is your God now?" I can assure you, He is there, in all of it. He won't always give you what you want, but He will give you what you need, when you put your trust and faith in Him.

> *For I know the plans I have for you, plans to prosper you and not harm you, plans to give you hope and a future. (Jeremiah 29:11)*

Life— it is tough at times, and honestly I don't know how people can get through this life without having faith in God. For me, He is my refuge and strength, through the good times and the bad.

Sometimes life's problems even seem to go from bad to worse. God is the only one who can reverse that downward spiral. He can take our problems and turn them into glorious victories if we just place our hope and trust in Him. The first step is we have to have faith, and be willing to turn *to* Him, even if we have doubts in what we cannot see, but we still must just trust in Him alone.

Many times we don't turn to God because our life is going great with us at the helm. We don't see God, and we don't seem to need God, so why fix something if it's not broken? In fact, it is at times like that when it's easy to forget that God actually created us, and put the breath in our lungs. But the truth is, we need to have faith in God *before* the storms come. Because if we can't trust that God is there in the little things, we won't be able to hold up when the big storms of life come.

My faith has grown stronger at various times of pain and despair in my life. There have been many highs and lows in my life. But nothing affected me more than losing my dad, my dear sister Arlene, and then my precious Mom. If you have never witnessed someone close to you leaving this life, you have no idea how it changes you deep in your core. We only have one family, one Mom and one Dad. To see all three of them take their last breath was something I will never forget. All three times, the deep and painful loss felt like more than I thought I could bear, but yet, as strange as it may seem, I had peace that surpassed all understanding afterwards, even mine. That was the Holy Spirit giving me peace, because it was certainly something I couldn't even comprehend. Only God.

God's Word tells us that He will give us that peace when we know Him and believe in His sovereignty. This is truth.

As I look back, it amazes me that I had the incredible opportunity to lead each of my family members to accept Christ as their Savior, and then to escort each of them out of this world with my hand in their hand, as they transitioned. I didn't plan that, God did. He had me there exactly at the right time. And I know now that their lives didn't end, they only changed—and for the better! God took them, and I had to look beyond earth's shadows into what I could not see and trust in the Lord our God with faith that *His* will was done.

Without having faith in God, I don't know how I could have endured the loss. Somehow I knew that if my father, sister and mother lived, that God didn't make a mistake. And I knew if He took them home to Heaven, that God didn't make a mistake. He took them for His Kingdom, and they are all pain-free, happy, joyful and at peace with God in Heaven! How can I be sad about that? Yes, I miss them in my life now more than words can say, but I *know* I will see them again.

Peace—the kind that surpasses all understanding. When we seek God first in everything we do, and we trust in His sovereignty, and we walk by faith, He will not allow us to be shaken no matter if the "sky is falling" or not. In fact I can lean into the storms now, and know that I am safe. I am not afraid to die because I know where I am going. And I am content to live without some of my family members because I know where they are and who they are with. Only God.

I miss my family, yes, and I do have my moments. I understand that my loss is Heaven's gain. In the meantime I continue to have faith, and trust God our Father, and I am so grateful for the opportunity to witness to all three of them the way I did. How many people have the opportunity to lead their father, mother and sister to Christ? That was not from something great I made happen, it was really God using me in ways I never imagined, for *His* glory, and for *His* kingdom, and I am so grateful for that.

Life here must go on and let's face it, it is tough at times. If you are struggling with health issues, family issues, or food issues, or you want to lose weight, gain weight, save your marriage, get married, have a baby, save your loved ones, or whatever it is you are trying to do, you need to seek God first, and have faith in God our creator!

We first have to believe that we are worthy of being healthy, and happy, and living that abundant life God desires for us. Then to get there, we also need to believe and truly understand that we can do all things through Christ alone who strengthens us, walking by faith. We need to have faith and trust Him, even when it doesn't make sense!

> *Trust in the Lord with all your heart, and lean not on your own understanding. In all ways acknowledge Him and He will make your paths straight. (Proverbs 3:5-6)*

I have experienced that faith firsthand in my life over and over. God did give me the desires of my heart many times when I thought nothing was possible. He is sovereign and His Word is truth. His ways are incomprehensible. God's sovereignty and His wisdom are things we can't even wrap our heads around. He has supernatural power, and He knows what we need before we even ask for it. Did you ever try and tell God what you need? Listen, He knows your needs—He's God! Just pray and lay your burdens down.

God himself says in Isaiah 55:8-9:

> *"For my thoughts are not your thoughts, neither are your ways my ways," declares the Lord. "As the Heavens are higher than the earth, so are my ways higher than your ways and my thoughts higher than your thoughts."*

Nothing is too big or too trivial for God. The one who created the universe and everything in it, including us, loves us, believes in us, and thinks we are very significant! How wild is that? Besides that, God knit us together in our mother's womb, and He knows how many hairs we have on our head. He holds the universe together hour by hour. He sustains what He creates. And when you really start seeking Him first, *He* will direct your paths and open your eyes like you never imagined. His Word even tells us that all we need is a mustard seed of faith. Did you know that the word "faith" appears in the Bible 458 times? There is a reason for that!

This I know for sure:

God is who He says He is.
God is Sovereign.
God is infinite in wisdom.
God is Love.

Have doubts? Read the Bible! Those pages and God's Word will come to life before your eyes. Pray beforehand, that God speaks to you so that you understand His words and commandments.

Everything we need to know about life and death and everything in between is in the Bible! In fact I love looking at the word Bible as an acronym meaning "Basic Instructions Before Leaving Earth." Everything we need to know is in this life manual, if we would only take the time to read it and allow the Holy Spirit to speak to us! Until you do that, it's not going to make sense. We wouldn't operate an important or dangerous piece of equipment without reading the manual cover to cover. Why wouldn't we read the BIBLE that contains the words of our Creator cover to cover?

5

Here's the thing: God made our body and mind one, and we know that when you have a healthy mind, you have a better chance of having a healthy body, and vice versa! But your spiritual life has to be healthy as well. The outside of your body can look okay, but your soul could be starving, creating an imbalance of your entire temple.

Soul Neglect

My good friend Linda Penn, radio host of *Today's Living Hope* on WDCX Christian radio, teaches that there are several signs of Soul Neglect:

1. Low-grade depression.
2. Busy but bored.
3. Loss of control over life's routine.
4. Loss of responsiveness to others.
5. Withdrawal from responsibility and leadership.
6. Preoccupation with projects of lesser importance/procrastination.
7. Resurgence of unhealthy habits, diminished impulse control, and diminished resistance to temptation.
8. Shame and guilt.
9. A hardened heart/rebellion due to hurt, pain, divorce, rape, loss of a loved one, or other circumstances.

Linda says, "As there are consequences to our health, there are consequences to our soul neglect."

1. When our souls need attention, we satisfy the wrong appetite. We misread the inner discomfort we feel and do the opposite.
2. We yield to temptation. That is a powerful source of destruction.
3. Deliberate sin shrinks the soul, wringing vitality from it. It lowers our immune system. We can become physically, emotionally, and spiritually sick.

Man was made for God, and man will never find happiness until he finds it in the One who made him.
—Saint Augustine

We have a tape recording in our heads, playing and replaying all day long. You may believe wrong thoughts, lies; you begin to justify, defend, or blame yourself. With unresolved conflict we begin to be defensive, angry at others, and act out. Soon we are self-destructing.

So, you are at a crossroads and you have a decision to make. Who am I going to follow? Is it Jesus, with a surrendered life to Him, or the other path, which only leads to destruction?

There is hope for healing. No matter what has happened to you in your life, or what you think, there is hope in Christ.

Rejection, abandonment, neglect, emotional, physical, sexual or spiritual abuse, difficulty in relationships, loss of loved ones, abortion, wrong decisions, criminal activity, rejecting God, participating in evil or wickedness, death, adultery, or illness, it doesn't matter. There is hope and a plan for your life. Read the Bible, go to church, get involved with others to grow and learn to have a healthy soul, and stay on track.

To know God, you need to commit or renew your relationship with Him by slowing down, resting, praying, and listening to find that sweet intimacy with Him. Our lives are about "being with Him," not just "doing life with Him."

I pray that you may prosper in every way and be in good health, just as your soul prospers. (3 John 2)

God's desire for our life is clear in the scripture but how do we start? Well, first and foremost we have to take our hands off the wheel, get rid of our pride, and realize that we *need* Jesus! Did you know that we go through trials and tribulations in our lives to grow deeper in our faith? And everyone goes through them, by the way. It's not a matter of **if** those trials and tribulations will come, it's **when** they will come. We need to be prepared to lean into the storm, and trust in God our Father. Suffering will happen, but it reminds us of Christ's suffering on the Cross, which was the greatest sacrifice of all. Jesus died so we could live.

You know, I had read the Bible earlier in my life, and gone to church, but I never really "got anything out of it." I didn't understand what the priest and pastors were saying, and I didn't understand the Bible. It was all Greek to me. But I knew that the people in my life who really "knew God" had something I didn't have. They had peace, joy, and stability, no matter

7

what life threw at them. I didn't have that, and I wanted it. Life was getting complicated and stressful. I was buckling under the pressure, and a lot of things were going wrong at the time. I was searching for happiness but no matter what I did—I couldn't find it.

So I prayed and prayed and even asked God to give me the words to pray, since I didn't know what to say or what to ask for. Fortunately God used someone to speak into my life, on the radio no less, and I committed myself to the Lord, even though at that time I didn't really understand fully what that even meant. That someone was Neil Boron, radio host at WDCX. He affected me in a profound way over the airwaves, and I had never even met him. This was many years ago, but I will never forget it.

I'm going to be honest, I always believed in God, and committed and recommitted to following Him several times. But there were times in my life when I wondered where He was, and I felt very lost and alone. Here I was on top of the world in so many ways, but yet something was very wrong and very missing in my life, and I felt this constant tug at my heart. I was actually on sinking sand, but at the time didn't know it. I would draw close to God, but then backslide. Then one day, while teaching classes and working in Manhattan, right in the middle of Times Square, God spoke right into my life, and really *saved* my life. That day, I was praying that God would just take over my life in every way, shape and form, and He did just that, in an unbelievable way.

This was the defining point in my life, where I made the decision that I was going to live my life for God alone, and I was *not* turning back. Tears were running down my face, and in that very moment, although I didn't realize the gravity of it at the time, my life was completely transformed by the Holy Spirit, and I am so grateful for that. There is no turning back for me now, and God is still transforming me every day, because we are all imperfect human beings, only He is perfect. But God dwells inside me, I love Him, and I have decided to follow Him – forever, no matter what.

Make the decision to spend time with God; spend time in His Word during the good times and bad. Listen to what He has to say, pray, ask Him to take over your life, and don't forget to thank Him for the blessings. He sees our heart, He knows when we are rebellious, and He knows when we are tracking with Him. He wants to transform us through the Holy Spirit, and He will, if you ask Him. But He won't force himself on us, because He gives us free will.

So, as fate would have it, not only was I saved by God's grace, but then God placed me on the same airwaves where I first felt the tug at my heart, on WDCX some twenty plus years later with my own show *The Raw Truth*. And I also had the opportunity to help Neil Boron lose fifty-plus pounds and get in shape with my Raw Truth Recharge! Was all this a coincidence? I think not. God obviously had a plan for my life, and He has one for your life too!

When you feel God is pulling at your heartstrings and you just continue to try and steer your life in the direction **you** think it should go instead of listening to Him, sooner or later He will just grab your heart, and He will stop you right in your tracks. That's what happened to me, and I'm so thankful it did.

So I went from wondering where God was in my life to now seeing His hand in everything. I am in the Word daily, sometimes several times a day, and miraculously He does speak to me often. Not audibly—it's hard to explain, but I know He's speaking. God speaks to me through Pastor Jerry Gillis, my pastor at The Chapel at CrossPoint, and through many other pastors and friends God has placed in my life. I am hungry for what God is teaching, and to experience how He is transforming me every day. But it took that first step of faith of "letting go and letting God," to start seeing the work God is doing in my life.

Faith can move mountains.

> *God's Word tells us if we have faith the size of a mustard seed, you could say to this mountain, "Move from here to there," and it will move. (Matthew 17:20)*

What I have noticed in my practice is that people are struggling in whatever it is they are trying to do, because they are trying to accomplish things based on their own great works. No matter what they are struggling with in their life, or whatever it is they are trying to achieve, people try to control the path of their life, and many don't look to God for answers or direction. Remember, I was there, and I can relate.

Listen, if you don't remember anything else in this chapter, remember this: life can and will be challenging. You will go through trials and tribulations in life, and the only way you can get through is by faith. And you later find out that those trials make your faith grow deeper, and you learn that God can give you the supernatural ability to persevere in the midst of the storm.

> *Consider it pure joy, whenever you face trials of many kinds, because you know that the testing of your faith develops perseverance. (James 1:2)*

Faith in God changes everything. When you have faith, God will breathe new life into your dreams. Faith puts feet to our prayers! Faith may not remove our problems but it gives us strength to lean into the storm and withstand our trials, and just trust in His sovereignty no matter what happens. Worry ends when faith in God begins, and peace is the result. I can still have peace and joy in the midst of my grief in losing my family, because I know God is sovereign.

Did you know that a growing number of medical and psychological studies have shown that spirituality, faith in God, and prayer have a definite positive impact on people's well-being, both physically and psychologically? It's no surprise that trust and belief in a loving God, prayer and meditation, attendance to regular Bible studies and fellowship with other believers have been shown to lead to improved physical and mental health, including lower levels of worry, stress, depression, suicide, and destructive behavior. People who believe in something greater than themselves are generally happier and healthier people according to the research. Of course it has also been shown that faith in God can give a person a more positive mental outlook that can significantly help their recovery from illness and surgery. No surprise there.

Any time we demonstrate faith, we're relying on something outside ourselves. Faith in God means we rely on Him, on who He is, and His sovereignty. It means believing that God is greater than our circumstance, and that He is sovereign, and He is! He is God.

There are many unknowns in life but sometimes we have to let go completely before God will work it all out, work through us, and within us. Stop struggling to take your hands off the wheel, and allow God to take control of your life and circumstances. He's got this! He made us, but we sometimes believe we have a better plan than the one who created us, the universe, and everything in it! That's pretty crazy when you think about it. It doesn't even sound logical. Maybe it's pride; maybe it's that we don't

10

trust God because we can't see Him. We want to use our logic, our smarts, our education, our science to get what we think we need. But again, God created us, the universe, and everything in it! And if you have any doubts, ask Him to come into your life and show you He's real. He will.

God's Word says we have not because we ask not. So you must *ask, seek, and knock* before the door will be opened. God won't force himself on us. He gave us free will to make our own decisions. Ask Him, and do it with faith, and then believe He will answer. He will, I tell you.

> *But let him ask in faith, nothing wavering. For he that wavers is like a wave of the sea driven with the wind and tossed. (James 1:6)*

We were made to glorify and honor God and bring others to Him. So we just need to walk by faith, even when you cannot see. We need to glorify Him with our actions and life, serve others, and bring others to know Him. He will bless us for that. Look at it this way, Jesus died for us. I think we can go out on a limb for Him and believe *in* Him!

We were saved by grace, and God's Word tells us:

> *For it is by grace you have been saved, through faith, and this not from yourselves, it is the gift from God. (Ephesians 2:8)*

If you are struggling, or even if you're not, have faith. What do you have to lose? Are you afraid of what you might find? Are you afraid of failing? The key to fear of failure is faith. Have some faith in God and His ability to deliver you the exact lessons you need to grow and become whole.

Remember that God has perfect timing; never early, never late. It takes a little patience and faith, but it's worth the wait—just ask Him!

First, ask God to come into your heart and take over your life in thought, in words, in actions. Lay down your pride and say "I need you, God, and if you are there please reveal yourself to me! I can't do this alone any more; I need you to take the helm. I want eternal life with you, Lord. Come into my heart and take over my life, Lord. I love you. ."

Faith is not the belief that God will do what you *want*. It is the belief that God will do what you *need*. As God's Word does tell us:

Whenever you ask for in prayer with faith, you will receive. (Matthew 21:22)

His promise is true, and He will never forsake us. Never stop praying, no matter how dark and hopeless it may seem. Keep your faith.

Having faith is different from having understanding. When you don't understand, trust that God is still at work! Faith isn't believing that God *can*; it is believing that God *will*.

If you are trying to eat healthy, lose weight, gain weight, reverse your disease, whatever it is, know that our flesh is lazy. Our flesh has no self-control. We first have to believe we can do all things—and we can. Commit to the Lord, then *trust* God's plan that He will not harm you, but that He will help you, even when it doesn't make sense. Pastor Jerry Gillis explained it this way, "to surrender to God is not weakness, it's a weapon."

Commit to the Lord whatever you do, and your plans will succeed. (Proverbs 16:3)

Trust in the Lord with all your heart; lean not on your own understanding. In all your ways acknowledge Him and He will direct your paths. (Proverbs 3:6)

Along with faith, we have to have *hope* that our needs will be met. The biblical definition of *hope* is "confident expectation."

Hope is a firm assurance regarding things that are unknown and unseen. Without hope, life loses its meaning. The righteous who trust or put their hope in God will be helped. (Psalm 28:7)

Those who have this trustful hope in God have a general confidence in God's protection and help; that He has a plan for us; that He wants us to prosper and not to harm us.

With all this said, I get that many of you are reading this book to achieve better health and fitness. Do you want to stop overindulging in food? *Do you want to get lean? Then lean on the Lord!*

God made our body and mind one—and a healthy mind leads to a healthy body! Today and every day, ask God to give you strength and self-control to resist the bad foods that cause disease. Focus on all the foods of the earth that God has supplied for us to fuel and feed our bodies—the nutrient-dense foods, the ones you don't need to read a label on, the ones that come from the earth.

What better day than today to start eating better and taking care of the "mobile home" God gave you? Everything is a decision. Start by:

1) Asking God to renew your mind and then say, "I am able" with God. "I am able to do whatever I need to do through Christ who strengthens me. "
2) Look away from those things that distract you. Change your focus from food to God and pray for strength and self-control. Stay in the Word daily!
3) Put a Post-it note on your refrigerator that says, "'We can do this together, I am with you and for you' – Love, God." And know you are worth it!

Only 10% of how we live is dictated by our genes. Ninety percent is dictated by our lifestyle habits. That's important to know, but what's even more important than living well on this planet is knowing God well. Before we can reach our fitness and health goals, or accomplish anything, we need God, and we need to have faith and hope.

To have health, wellness, and fitness, it doesn't matter where you start—it just matters that you *do* start! And when you do start, know you are not alone on this journey as God is with us and for us. Have faith that:

We can do all things through Christ who strengthens us.
(Philippians 4:13)

Be confident in knowing that God wants us to take care of our bodies:

Do you not know that your body is a temple of the Holy Spirit,
who is in you, whom you have received from God? You are not
your own; you were bought at a price. Therefore honor God
with your body. (1 Cor. 6:19-20)

Those of us who are followers of Christ know that our life is better because we believe in Jesus and follow Him, rather than trying to accomplish things on our own accord—we can have faith in Him alone, no matter what happens. God is in control, and that takes a lot of pressure off! That doesn't mean, by the way, that your life will be perfect once you decide to follow God, it just means you will have peace in knowing He is sovereign.

I don't know about you, but I pray to God several times a day. I have my morning and evening quiet time when I am deliberate about reading God's Word and praying, but there are also several times throughout the day that I am talking to Him, thanking Him, and praying. Pastor Jerry Gillis says, "Pray to obey, not to get your way" – His will not ours.

Pray without ceasing. (1 Thessalonians 5:16-18)

I'm telling you this because I have faith that God is listening to my prayers and will answer them if it's His will, and He has proved that. God has a way of reminding us that with Him all things are possible. God's Word doesn't say "some" things are possible—it says "*all things*" are possible with Christ. Give God all of your burdens!

Thank God today for the breath in your lungs, the beat of your heart... and LIVE the life God gave you to its fullest, with health, energy, and vibrancy. And no longer be sick, thick, and tired! Ask God to heal you of your disease and ailments. He hears you and knows your thoughts.

God longs to comfort us, lead us, and give us rest, no matter the magnitude of our struggle; in fact, He delights in it! And when we ask Him to come into our heart, and we lay our burdens at His feet, it's amazing how much peace we have no matter what our circumstances are. His Word is true, He will give you the desires of your heart, but will not harm you, or allow any wish you have for your life to harm you. Pray for His will not yours. Trust God, believe it, and receive it! Matthew 21:22 records Jesus's words, which teach that in all things that we pray for, we should believe to receive.

James 4:2 says we don't have, because we don't ask. I think many Christians today view sickness and illness as either mental or physical, as something they have no power to overcome, apart from doctors' appointments and drugstores. The Word of God teaches us that we have greater authority than most of us realize.

When you follow God's plan for your life you will reap the rewards of an abundant life in your health.

Remember that God is our only source of hope, and there are several awesome consequences of having hope in God. Here are a few, though there are so many more:

1 Timothy 4:10 – increased energy and passion
Philippians 1:20 – confidence
Romans 12:12 – joy through testing
Colossians 1:4-5 – greater faith and love
Romans 8:24-25 – perseverance
Hebrews 6:19 – security

When in doubt know these truths:

You say: It's impossible.
God says: *All things are possible.* (Luke 18:27)

You say: I can't figure it out.
God says: *I will direct your steps.* (Proverbs 3:5-6)

You say: I'm too tired.
God says: *I will give you rest.* (Matthew 11:28-30)

You say: I feel alone.
God says: *I will never leave you or forsake you.* (Hebrews 13:5)

You say: I am afraid.
God says: *I have not given you fear.* (2 Timothy 1:7)

You say: I can't manage.
God says: *I will supply all of your needs.* (Philippians 4:19)

You say: I can't do it.

God says: *You can do all things through Christ who strengthens you.* (Philippians 4:13)

You say: I can't go on.
God says: *My grace is sufficient for you.* (2 Corinthians 12:9)

You say: I can't forgive myself.
God says: *I forgive you.* (Romans 8:1)

You say: It's not worth it.
God says: *It will be worth it.* (Romans 8:28)

You say: I'm not smart enough.
God says: *I will give you wisdom.* (1 Corinthians 1:30)

You say: I am not able.
God says: *I am able.* (2 Corinthians 9:8)

You say: No one loves me.
God says: *I love you and proved it.* (John 3:16)

> *For those who live according to the flesh set their minds on the things of the flesh, but those who live according to the Spirit set their minds on the things of the Spirit. (Romans 8:5)*

Here's the truth: when we sin or when we aren't aligned with God and His will for our life, we are holding ourselves back from all the blessings He has for us. Just surrender and you will see His hand in your life, everywhere.

7 Truths To Help You On Your Faith Journey:

1) Stay in the Word daily and pray, even if it's just for five to ten minutes a day to start. Give thanks to God our Father first, and then lay your burdens down.
2) Remember that our purpose is to bring glory and honor to God. (1 Thessalonians 4:1)

3) Make a list of God's faithfulness and the blessings of your life at least once a month so you stay thankful and grateful. Count your blessings!

4) Remember that no matter what our circumstances or tests we are walking through, God will use it for His glory. Our tests will become our testimony. Our mess, our message.

5) Remember that God will never fail you. (Deuteronomy 31:6)

6) Believe it, conceive it, take steps to achieve it. Then leave the rest to God and prepare to receive it! Ask God to come into your heart and take over your life.

7) Be a light to others. If you are convicted in what you believe, you won't be able to hold back. Ask God to fill you with His Holy Spirit.

So here's the thing: as much as I care about my body, I also know that the condition of my heart is much more important to God than the "condition" of my body. What we think about God is the *most* important thing about us! And before we can reach our health and fitness goals, or accomplish anything – we need to believe, trust, and seek *Jesus*.

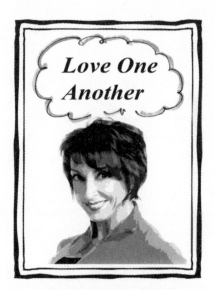

TRUTH TWO

Family – Love One Another

Y OU PROBABLY DON'T think much about the fact that a support system
and family are important to your mental and physical health. And,
you might not have chosen your family members, and sometimes you don't
understand them, but out of all the people on the planet, they're the ones
who are your blood and should love you unconditionally, and you should
love them back. They're the ones who cherish you, and whom you should
cherish in return.

Here's what I know: we can eat right and exercise all day long, but if
our relationships aren't healthy and we don't have that family support and
network, you won't be in a state of homeostasis, and really your life can be
toxic to your own health and well-being. Homeostasis is defined as a process
that maintains the stability of the human body's internal environment in
response to changes in external conditions. Without love and support from
your family and friends, your health, no matter how healthy you are, will
be affected both physically and mentally. We have an innate need to feel

loved, wanted, and accepted, and when we don't get that, we are starving at a level we are not even aware of.

"Vitamin L" is so important to your health and well-being. You may have never heard of this vitamin before, because it doesn't really exist in pill, isotonic form, or any other edible form for that matter. Of course I am talking about love. God wants us to love one another. Not only does He want us to love one another, His Word commands us to love one another several times in the Bible. For example:

> *Love one another. As I have loved you, so you must love one another. By this all men will know that you are my disciples, if you love one another. (John 13:34-35)*

God IS Love.
God's love is unreproducible.
God's love is unconditional.
God's love is unfathomable.
God's love is unfailing.
God's love is unending.

I learned the greatest love from my beautiful mother, her actions and words, and how she unselfishly loved me every day. When I think of God's love for us, I think of my mom. She was always there for me, and my prayer was that someday I would give that back tenfold to her.

I was brought up in a home that taught you should never let a day go by where you don't "show and tell" love to the people who are closest to you. Love is an action, and we need to be deliberate about it to demonstrate it.

My Dear Mom

Our primary goal in life should be to love, please, honor and glorify God, and others. My mom instilled that in me at an early age, and I was a witness to how love and family were so important. Consequently, to me, family and friends always signified love. No matter what happened in the world, I knew God loved me and I knew that my mom, family and close friends loved me.

Well as God would have it, I had the pleasure of taking care of my mom for twenty-plus years, and I am so grateful for that. It was my honor and pleasure to serve my mom. No matter what the weather, no matter what plans there were, I was there for Mom. There wasn't enough time in the day, but I made sure I'd carve out time for Mom.

My mom, the one who carried me in her womb, and sacrificed her entire life for me. The one who worked so hard every day at a job to provide for us, raised her family, and loved us kids like no other.

As Mom grew older, I cut down on my work and I was there morning, noon, and night. After all, I was always very aware of the fact that someday she would be gone, like my dad and sister. And I wanted to help her *live* as long as she could. She had told me that she didn't want to be in a nursing home ever, nor did I want her to be. She used to say, "When I wanted Robbie to be a nurse, I didn't know that I would be her number one patient." She was definitely my number one!

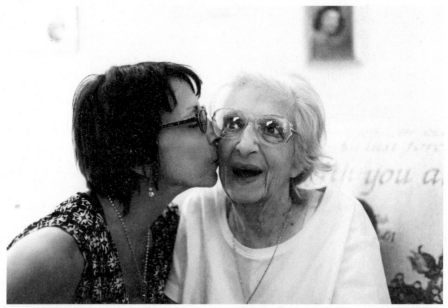

This picture was taken less than a month before Mom passed. I love it because the complete and utter look of joy on her face is what I suspect Mom had when she rose up on eagles' wings, and saw Jesus for the first time.

I remember taking Mom to the doctor when she was 80. Mom had been on twelve different medications over the years. You know, when you are on medication, you have to take other medication to counteract the side effects of the first medication, and it's a vicious cycle.

Mom had high blood pressure, high cholesterol, diabetes, and chronic obstructive pulmonary disease at this point in her life, and of course with all that, she was headed for a stroke. One day, I took Mom to see her favorite doctor and told him, "I would like to take over my mom's health care and get her off of these medications by changing her diet. Would you help me get towards that goal?" The doctor looked me straight in the eyes with a big smile and said, "Robbie, your mom is 80 years old, let her eat what she wants and give her medication."

Oh boy… he had no idea who he was talking to. I had to leave the room right then in an effort not to say something I would regret, and I went out to the desk and requested my mom's medical records that very day.

When Mom passed at the age of 92, she was off all medication except for one. I took her to the chiropractor weekly and for regular massages up until the week she passed away. And at 92, she was living in our home drinking green smoothies and eating organic food daily, with an occasional cannoli or rice pudding when she wanted it! Because at 92, if you want a cannoli you should have it! Mom was healthy as could be up until a month before she passed, when she started to decline.

Now I realize not everyone has the opportunity or knowledge to take care of his or her loved ones, but as a nurse, and because I had taken care of her for twenty years prior, I wasn't going to have it any other way. I honored her wishes as well, and I have no regrets.

I'd like to share some intimate and personal moments about my family in the hope that it will help you in your walk with God, because I am living proof that God carries us when we can't walk ourselves. God's Word tells us not only to love one another but also to carry each other's burdens.

I learned so much from my mom, which I will share with you here, because her wisdom and love were amazing, and I value what she taught me every day of my life, even now.

It was during the writing of this book, that my best friend, my dear Mom, went home to be with the Lord. Mom lived with us for the last year of her life, and she passed away in our home. I had been her sole caretaker for many years. Those final years were by far the most beautiful and precious moments of my life. You will never ever regret what you gave up to make time with loved ones. Because once they are gone, they are gone, and you miss them more than you can imagine.

Mom, the one who loved me more than anyone, aside from God. The unconditional love that no one but a mother or father has. The love and loss is so deep, sometimes it's more than I can stand, yet I know Mom is in Heaven and that her life has not ended, it has only changed, and actually has only just begun. I am so grateful that this isn't all there is!

You learn so much from people who have lived a long, hard life. Mom had lived through the Depression and raised us kids, for many years alone. I really don't know how she did it. She always had wisdom and discernment, and she always gave me advice whether I wanted it or not. She was giving me advice up to the week she passed away! We talked about everything and we shared everything. She was a great listener as well.

One of the things I recall about Mom's life struck me at the end: during her years, she was always counting her money in her change purse a couple of times a day! Mom was so thrifty. But in those final months of her life, she was not interested in her things, or in counting the money in her change purse anymore. In fact, she wouldn't even look in her purse those final months, even when I handed it to her. What she did do is stare at all the family photos on her dresser, especially the last few weeks of her life. When I would ask Mom why she kept staring at the pictures, she replied that she was trying to figure out why some people were missing now that had been in the pictures before.

Did she mean her daughter, or her sister, or her mother who were all in Heaven? I don't know, and she didn't say. Although I did tell her that they were in Heaven, she just kept staring. It is profound to think about those moments and how her priorities changed, in those final days, from her things to her loves.

Those final days were tough.

I had been praying for years for three things of which God actually gave me the desires of my heart:

1) That Mom would not suffer a stroke or anything like that, leaving her suffering in her final days. God answered my prayers, and she didn't suffer.
2) That I would always be able to take care of her and escort her out of this world. I did, until she passed.
3) And that when the Lord took her, I would be at her side holding her and comforting her (as I was with my Dad and my sister). I was.

As I looked back in the last few years and months of my mom's life, I saw God's hand in all of it. He answered my three prayers and gave me the desires of my heart, and it was not a coincidence.

It was April, and Mom wanted to go to Florida with the girls the way we had every year for decades. I was concerned about traveling with Mom this year, as she seemed to be fading. But after her doctors gave her the okay and said to me, "Robbie, go and create memories," I decided to take her. We boarded the plane and had the most memorable vacation I could ever remember. I fully recall thinking "this will be Mom's last trip." We captured some beautiful pictures of us by the ocean that I will cherish forever. I was so thankful to have that last vacation with Mom.

Easter came and went, and I had a huge birthday bash for Mom's ninety-second birthday on April 26th. All of her living siblings, nieces, nephews, and grandchildren were at our home to celebrate. I hired a professional photographer to capture the precious moments, and Mom was so happy.

The next family event was on May 30th, which is both my birthday and my sister Susan's—we are not twins, but we were born on the same day.

Mom always remembered our birthdays, of course, and everyone else's on the planet as well. But that morning I said to Mom "It's our birthday, Mom—Susan and I! Let's call Susan up and wish her a Happy Birthday!" Mom looked at me with a blank look and then said, "I don't know even know what you're talking about." I knew right then and there I was losing Mom fast. I replied with a huge lump in my throat while holding back the tears, "That's okay, Mom, don't worry about it," and I went upstairs and bawled my eyes out. I knew it was a matter of time before I lost her completely.

A few weeks before Mom passed, she had not been talking much. I had always made a point of taking several pictures and videos of Mom daily, realizing that we would not have a warning sign when that last day would come. On one particular day, I encouraged her to say a few words to each of her grandchildren on video. She was so very weak that day, but determined to say some beautiful, loving words with all of her strength, and she did just that. I knew at that moment that my mom was fully aware of the fact that her time with us was short. I knew in my heart that she did not want to leave us. Mom would not give up easily, and I was not ready to say goodbye. Those pictures and videos would later become more precious, than I could ever imagine.

At this point, Mom would still perk up when her grandchildren came in. She loved her children and grandchildren more than life itself, and every day she would ask me if they ate! A typical grandmother! She was their Nannie, and the kids loved her.

I will always remember the Sunday before she passed. It was Father's Day in June. It was an absolutely beautiful day, 80 degrees, and the sun was shining. Mom was getting weaker; I could see it, and no way was I going to leave her even to run to the store. I suggested to my husband Jeff that he go with our daughters to the Allentown Art Festival, as we liked to do every year. The Allentown Art Festival was big in our family, as my father was an accomplished artist who presented at Allentown for many years. It was also the second-last place I had taken my dear sister Arlene, also an artist, before she passed.

So Jeff and our girls left, and it was just Mom and I as it had been so many other times before. Mom, my little buddy; I loved being with her, just her and me. That day, Mom wasn't talking or eating very much at all, which of course was concerning. I had made sure she had some cereal, and a little green blueberry smoothie for breakfast. Some pudding is all she wanted for lunch. Looking out of the window, she commented how beautiful it was outside. I asked her if she wanted to go for a walk outside in the wheelchair and she said, "Yes, that would be nice."

She was extremely weak, but I got her dressed and in the wheelchair, and somehow using my own strength lifted the wheelchair down the front step and out of the front door myself (usually Jeff lifted her out of the door).

I was determined to do it one way or another that day, as I was fully aware there were not many more moments like this with her. I always thought that about Mom, any time I took pictures, etc. I was aware of the fact that it may be the last picture I'd take of Mom, or the last time we did this or that.

Of course I took several pictures of the two of us that day and posted a picture on social media saying "I fully realize that this moment will not last forever; cherishing every minute with Mom." Little did I know God would take her exactly one week later.

I pushed her around the neighborhood a few times, and she said only two things: "It's beautiful out," and "I love you, Robbie." I fed her some ice cream, which she loved, as we watched the birds.

When it was time to get her in, I could not lift the chair over the step with her in it. I tried and tried but didn't have the strength myself. I ended up calling my friend Beth and her husband Mike over, and Mike lifted her into the house. That would be the last day Mom was outside or even up out of bed. It gives me chills to remember that day. From that night on, things began to change drastically, and I knew there was no turning back.

In those final days, the presence of God was felt in my house and in her room in ways I had never felt in my entire life. I talked a lot to Mom, knew she could hear me, but her words were few. Mom would perk up when my kids or my nieces or nephews came into the room, and then she would go quiet again. She loved her girls and grandchildren like no other. Family was her life.

I kept a journal and was posting occasionally to Facebook to let people know how Mom was. I had posted pictures of Mom on social media for years, and she had a huge fan base of people who were inspired by her! It was comforting to read the responses that people were praying for Mom and I during that long week. I was fully aware that Mom, my best friend, was slipping away. I was losing her—how could this be, and what was I going to do without her? It was too much to even comprehend.

To give you an idea of my pain and thoughts at this time, here are some excerpts from my journal and my postings on Facebook. I just had to hold on to my strength and trust in God:

June 16th 2014 – (journal entry)

Mom does not want to eat, and sleeps most of the time. Susan is sleeping over tonight. Mom isn't saying much, but she tells us she loves us and we keep telling her the same. I refuse to leave the room or her side. I'm not ready to lose her, but I know she will live forever. Death will not separate us from God and his love. God's words comfort me, but this is so hard.

June 17th 2014 – (journal entry)

She's slipping away. I can see it. Family and the grandchildren have all been in, Mom perks up when they come in, and her words are few. She is so very weak. She was reaching for Uncle John and Aunt Karen, but doesn't have much strength. Mom and I just held each other all night, but she's so weak. I'm clinging to Jesus. God is with us. We shall not fear. He will change our weak mortal bodies and make them like his own glorious body. Philippians 3:21

June 18ᵗʰ 2014 (journal entry)

Mom is slowly slipping away and I have not left her side. She keeps looking at me and then stares at the ceiling. Her words are few, but she says she loves us. We keep telling her how much I love her. When I asked her why she kept staring at the ceiling she slowly replied, "Because there's more answers than questions up there." Wow. How profound is that? I knew exactly what she meant. Mom instilled the belief in God in me at an early age, and I know her faith is strong. I believe she is half in this world and half in the other. I'm losing her... Even though I walk through the valley of the shadow of death, I will not fear, for you are with me; your rod and staff comfort me. Psalm 23:4

June 19ᵗʰ, 2014 (journal entry)

Family has been in and out. Our pastor came to visit and Mom perked right up. When he asked if she was feeling "okay" she replied that she was "better than anyone else in the room"—wow. This was her first complete sentence of the day, and how profound. She is on her way to see Jesus so I don't doubt that! I don't want to lose her...

June 20ᵗʰ 2014 (Facebook post)

Dear Friends and Family – I am reading all of your posts and it is most comforting to know your hearts, how much you care, and how you are praying. Mom is still with us but only some of the time as the Transition to Heaven continues. My family and I are surrounding her with love right in our home, she has incredible peace, and we are finding strength and hope in The Lord our God. We have worship music playing constantly, and the love is intense. Our pastors told us they could feel God's presence in our home and we are on sacred ground. I love that. Her life is not ending – It's only changing – for the better! As she will be in the arms of JESUS! Will keep you posted as we plan to celebrate her long beautiful life, which has touched so many of us in ways we can't describe. It's so overwhelming but I do find comfort in your notes and posts, and I know many of you have gone through this. God bless you all and thank you again. I love you all with God's love ~ Robbie

June 20ᵗʰ 2014 (journal entry)

Spending the night lying next to her and holding Mom. Her breathing is changing, and her pulse is weak. I am turning her every couple of hours. It's just her and I again, and we don't let go of one another. She still has not responded but I know she knows I am here. Worship music is on continuously as it gives us comfort. I know she can hear me so I am praying and talking to her, but there is no response.

June 21ˢᵗ 2014 (journal entry)

It was Saturday night, and I was lying in bed with Mom – her eyes were wide open staring at the ceiling as if she was watching something. All of a sudden with just Mom and I there in the dark of the night, Mom started reaching up toward the ceiling as if she was reaching for someone above the bed. I was so amazed at what I was seeing, I was shaking, but I happened to have my phone next to me and I started snapping photos of her reaching up.

As I was doing this, I said "Mom! Mom! Do you see Jesus?!" She then let out this squeak and I knew she was saying yes. I asked her again. "Mom! Do you see Jesus?!" And she once again squeaked! I know she heard me, and I know she saw Jesus. And I know she wanted me to know that. Her eyes were so big and she was focused. Let me tell you that prior to this, the days before this happened, she hadn't eaten for a week. Mom didn't even have enough strength to raise her baby finger, let alone her arm, but she was reaching up with her entire arm and hand, with full strength. Do I think she saw Jesus? – absolutely. I believe He was coming to get her. She would pass on several hours later the next day on Sunday, the Lord's day. I am clinging to Jesus.

June 22ⁿᵈ 2014 (journal entry)

I spent the night laying next to Mom and watching her all night. She is no longer responding or reacting. Her breathing has changed drastically now and the hospice was called. Our good friend Dr. Sam Shatkin came to see her in the early morning and we prayed for her. I am losing her quickly and I can't believe this is happening. I love you Mom…forever.

June 22ⁿᵈ 2014 (Facebook post)

Dearest Friends and Family,

Thank you all for your thoughts and prayers as they have comforted me so much over the past days, weeks, and months. My precious Mom took her FIRST breath in Heaven at 2:32 pm today on the Lord's Day! My daughter Shanelle, my sister Susan, and I held her hands on this side, and I know our heavenly sister Arlene and Jesus wrapped their arms around her in Heaven on that side. I will post information about the wake and funeral tomorrow and you are ALL welcome to celebrate her life with us the following days, as I know she has touched so many of us.

I am so glad that this world is not our home, and that God promises each of us everlasting life in Heaven. And when you know the Lord you realize that our death day is better than our Birthday! Absent from the body is present with The Lord! How awesome is that!

Please stay tuned for more details posted here tomorrow on the celebration of Theresa Palmisano – our amazing Mom! God Bless you all! And thank you again ~ Robbie

June 22, 2014 (journal entry)

Mom went into the arms of Jesus today at 2:32 pm. My heart is breaking but I have unexplainable peace that passes all understanding. Absent with the body – present with The Lord! I don't need to pray for her anymore but I know she is still praying for us. I still feel her with me and I know I will see her again and we will pick up where we left off when she was "young and healthy." The pain is deep, but I know Mom is healthy and in Heaven, she is better than us! No more pain. I love you forever Mom, and I will miss you until I see you again.

Mom's funeral was a beautiful celebration of her long life. I gave the eulogy and I knew she didn't want me up there crying. Pastor Jerry Gillis performed the ceremony. Mom loved The Chapel at CrossPoint, and always said she loved Pastor Jerry. And at 92, she even commented on how handsome he was! She used to see him up there on the pulpit and say, "Is he the one I like?"

At Mom's beautiful celebration, Neil Boron, Jill Kelly, and I spoke about our memories of Mom and what kind of person she was. There was beautiful worship music, and Pastor Jerry Gillis gave us words of comfort.

Those days will be etched in my mind forever, my fingers enlaced with my mom's until the very end. I never left my mom's side. I was able to escort my mom from this world to the next with all the love and respect I could possibly give her. The hospice and the pastors told me they never saw such love. I was just trying to give back the love I had felt from Mom all those years. When she took her last breath, amazingly I had peace that surpasses all understanding—even mine. It was supernatural.

I urge you to spend the time with your parents and loved ones now before they are gone. When they are gone, they are gone. Show them you love them. I have no regrets spending time with my mom, dad and sister, and I would do it all over again if I had the chance. The other stuff will always be there, but don't miss the time now while you have it with those that matter. And no matter what happens, remember that when we accept Christ as our Savior, He gives us eternal life – and we will soon receive an incorruptible body and be present with the Lord.

I love Jeremy Camp's song "There Will Be a Day."

> *There will be a day with no more tears, no more pain, and no more fears*
> *There will be a day when the burdens of this place, will be no more, we'll see Jesus face to face*
> *But until that day, we'll hold on to you always*

God's Word gave me so much peace, knowing:

> *"Our Citizenship is in Heaven" (Philippians 3:20)*

> *"He who believes in me shall never die" (John 11:25-27)*

> *"Death does not conquer those who die in Christ" (Corinthians 15:22 53-56)*

> *"God is our refuge and strength, an ever-present help in trouble" (Psalm 46:1)*

> *"Even though I walk through the valley of the shadow of death, I shall fear no evil. For you are with me; your rod and your staff, they comfort me." (Psalm 23:4)*

> *"Be still and know that I am God" (Psalm 46:10)*

God gives me peace and joy and all the things I need. And my mom's wisdom taught me so much in her ninety-two years. She gave me advice and told me what to do up to the week she passed. I will never forget the top twenty things my mom instilled in me that I hope to remember forever:

1) Pray about everything. Go to church and believe in God. He loves you and so do I.
2) Love your sisters. Friends may come and go but sisters will always be your sisters, even in Heaven.
3) Always be there for your family and friends and carry each other's burdens.
4) Always be honest and tell the truth.
5) Forgive and forget.
6) Count your blessings.
7) Never burn bridges.
8) Love one another deeply.
9) Hold on to your good friends.
10) Give more than you take (she demonstrated this every day).
11) Remember I love you, and be sure to love your children. You can't love too much.
12) Make your bed when you get up—it takes up 80% of the room.
13) Eat your vegetables! (See where I get it from?)
14) Keep your room, and your house, clean. And no clothes on the floor!
15) Use your manners.
16) Put your feet down.
17) Respect your elders.
18) Don't be a cream puff (meaning stay strong)!
19) Work hard, but have fun.
20) Eat, eat, eat—before you get sick, or when you are sick, and for every and any reason—just EAT. You'll feel better.

Words of the wise that I hope to pass on for generations to come.

Those lessons from Mom will stay with me forever. She always made the best of every situation and encouraged me to do the same. This verse reminds me of what she taught me.

Finally, brothers and sisters, whatever is true, whatever is noble, whatever is right, whatever is pure, whatever is lovely, whatever is admirable—if anything is excellent or praiseworthy—think about such things. (Philippians 4:8)

My Dear Sister Arlene

My world was rocked and my faith grew deep when my dear sister Arlene's life was changed forever. Arlene and I loved to shop, hang out, fly back and forth to New York, go to Toronto together, go to the beach, the show, go on cruises together, and do everything sisters do. Our kids were around the same age, and her kids were like my own kids, and we did a lot together with the children as well.

I was on my honeymoon in Cancun, and my husband and I were just coming in from the beach when we found out from the front desk there had been a call to the hotel from my sister and it was important. I thought, "Wow, that's weird that my sister would be calling me the first day of my honeymoon." I knew before I called her back that something was wrong. It was then I learned that Arlene had breast cancer. We had both worked for the same doctor, a doctor we trusted. She had been told she had a blocked milk duct by the doctor, our boss and friend, and we believed that. We had no reason to think anything else. She had been pregnant two years in a row, and we had no history of breast cancer in our family. It didn't even cross our minds.

I was in shock at first. We all were. How could she have been misdiagnosed for two years with what doctors thought was a blocked milk duct? How could that happen? How could we have missed this ourselves? When Arlene was rightly diagnosed at the age of 42, she had four sons, two of them new babies to care for, and she was given only a few years to live with what was then diagnosed as Stage 4 breast cancer. Hearing world-class doctors tell you something like that, I think most people would give up or think their life was over. Not my sister, and not me. I told my sister back then, and I will say with all confidence now, that with all due respect to the doctors I know and those I don't know, they are not God. No one knows the day and the hour of our death, except for God.

Arlene was a wonderful mom and principal who loved her own children more than life itself and loved her kids at school. She was a fighter. What transpired over the years following was a true miracle, a story of

God's incredible grace, a will to *live*, being your own health advocate, and having awesome faith in God—because she actually lived ten years past her diagnosis. It was at that time that my focus changed from fitness to health, and I researched the link between cancer and diet. What kept standing out in the research was the link between sugar and dairy and breast cancer. I began to learn about cancer-fighting foods and nutritional holistic therapies at that time, and bought my sister a juicer back in the days when most people never thought of juicing.

As most people woke up every day and went on with their lives, I watched my sister fight for her life with the most positive attitude and faith in God I had ever seen. My mom and I took Arlene to every appointment, treatment, and test. Through the many surgeries, hospitalizations, chemotherapy, radiation, gamma knife treatments, and experimental treatments, she walked through the valley of death and fought a courageous battle with an incredible faith in God and a will to live like no other.

Those ten years were unbelievable. And her boys, her husband, and my family cherished every day we had her. We did everything together as we did before. We took our kids to the beach, went on trips, went on cruises together with Mom and the kids. Arlene had a strong faith, and as with my mother and my father we had many talks about God and eternal life. We prayed together many times, and like Mom and Dad, she accepted Christ as her Savior, a year before she passed. Thanks be to God!

I have a lot of beautiful memories of Arlene over those last ten years, but fast-forward to the final months and days. I had many cherished conversations with my sister in the last months, days, and hours of her life.

Arlene was dedicated to her family and boys. I clearly remember one of the many times she and I had been in New York City for an appointment at Sloan Kettering Hospital, and she had a bandage on her head from her recent brain treatments. She was weak and not well, but she was determined, and she proceeded to drag us all over the city to try and get a beautiful cross necklace for her son Christopher's First Communion. Arlene always put herself last and never complained or seemed to give in to the disease, although inside, I knew in my heart she was losing the fight.

Another time Arlene and I were going to NYC. I was taking her to Sloan Kettering Hospital for treatment, but I happened to pass out on the plane on the way there, due to hypotension. This had happened to me before on my way home from Las Vegas from a Fitness Conference. In fact the plane had to do an emergency landing in Kansas because they could not find my pulse! I then woke up on a stretcher and I thought we crashed! I thought everyone was on a stretcher, and I was thanking Jesus that I lived! I'm sure glad it wasn't a plane crash!

So, I passed out on the plane this time with Arlene, was carried off and into an ambulance with Arlene by my side. I then heard her ask the ambulance driver if they could take me to a hospital in Times Square, close to where we were staying. I was lying in the emergency room, while Arlene went to check into the hotel. Now I must say, Arlene was not doing that well, as the cancer was spreading.

But she had a great attitude, and along with her treatments, she wanted to make sure we did three things on this trip, shop, see a play, and go to Carnegie Hall. And trust me I was going to make sure she was able to do all three. So there I was, in the emergency room with intravenous fluids in my arm, and they were about to do some tests. The next thing I know Arlene comes in and says, "take those IV's out, we have tickets for Carnegie Hall!" And I thought to myself, my sister is dying and she wants to live life to it's fullest. I'm taking these IV's out, and we are going to Carnegie Hall! Although I don't recommend this, I took my IV out, signed myself out of the hospital and we had the most amazing time ever at Carnegie Hall. I will never forget that moment and how much Arlene wanted to enjoy life, every bit of it.

There were many other moments like this where Arlene did whatever she could no matter how sick she was, against all odds, to be there for her boys' games and their special events. Her will to live life to its fullest each day was more than many people have in a lifetime.

The last few months of my sister's life were tough. She was living at my mom's house where Mom and I could be her caretakers and do what we could 24/7. Her husband George was amazingly taking care of their four boys himself in their home. He did something that most fathers could not do in dedicating his life to those four boys, and training them up alone. I am grateful for him and consider him my blood brother rather than brother-in-law, and I feel the boys are like my own sons. I know how deeply my sister loved them all, and how proud she was of her boys.

Arlene was a principal, as I mentioned, and a few months before she passed, her school was closed due to downsizing. Arlene loved that school, her job, the staff, and the children there so much, and she was very upset to see it close. I think she knew in her heart she would never be returning, and this was a chapter of her book ending. A playground in Arlene's name and memory would later be dedicated to her.

Arlene was not eating much at all but loved Tim Horton's iced coffee, and every day either I would bring her one or my Aunt Helen would bring her one. Arlene was fading fast, but she was hanging on to every last bit of her life for her boys, and to see her son Keith's baby born, which was going to be any day. I had worship music playing in her room continuously, and at night I would sleep at my mom's and read her Scripture and devotions before bed.

Fifteen days before Arlene passed, on August 14th, we got the call that her beautiful grandchild Ashton was born. When we told Arlene, she sat right up in bed and said, "I'm going to the hospital."

Now mind you, she could barely stand up alone. Mom and I dressed Arlene together, and somehow we got her down the stairs of my mom's home, back in the wheelchair, and into my car. Arlene was so determined and excited that day, it was clear to me that she *lived* for this moment, and I will never forget it. Nor will I ever forget the first time she saw and held Ashton, her first grandchild. I cry just thinking about that moment. It was the most beautiful moment of my life, and most certainly hers.

The week before Arlene passed, George and the boys came to visit, as they did several times a week. She was too weak to get out of bed at this point, but still very aware of what was happening. I remember on this particular night, George walked into the bedroom, and my sister, lying in bed, said, "George, I can't do this anymore." I knew this was a turning point for Arlene, as she had always fought so hard to live.

The last week of my sister's life was awful, as I saw her young life slip away from this world. She was so young, and she had wanted to live for her boys so much. While writing these words I am crying, as the loss again is so deep and the pain is still there, for all of us. But in my heart, I know she is pain-free in Heaven in the arms of Jesus our Savior. Again, how can I be sad about that? I am just so glad this life is not all there is.

Two nights before Arlene passed, I was lying next to her on a rollaway bed, praying, reading the Bible, and watching her. In the middle of the night, she yelled out "Don't take me so far, don't take me so far!"

Her eyes were closed but I said "Arlene! Who are you talking to?" She replied "Dad." (He had passed a few years earlier). I said "Arlene, where are you?" She replied "On a path, on a runway." I said "Arlene, it's okay, follow that path and the light to Jesus. Jesus is coming for you—it's ok to let go." (As a nurse who has experienced the death of my patients many times, I am fully aware that they need to be told it's okay to go).

It was then in those final hours of her life, that I promised my sister two things:

1) To always be there for her four beautiful boys.
2) To fight to find a cure for breast cancer.

This was the last time she told me she loved me.

In our many talks, I knew both of those things were very important to her. And that's why I feel this has been part of my "calling" right now.

The night before Arlene passed, I was again lying next to her awake. In the middle of the night, my mom came into the room and said she had just heard Arlene call her. I said, "I have been right here, and she hasn't said anything at all." That was strange; Mom was convinced that Arlene yelled out to her.

The morning Arlene passed, her breathing was changed and rapid. She was not responding but looked peaceful and without pain. I called my brother-in-law and told him I thought today was going to be the day, and that he may want to get the two older boys out of school and come. Shortly after that, they were there by her side with my mom and me, and our sister Susan.

The hospice nurse had come in that morning, and I said to her, "I think today is the day." She said to me, "Oh no, I think she has a couple more days." It was only a few hours later that afternoon that God took Arlene to be with Him in Heaven. Her life, like my dad's and mom's, didn't end, it only changed—for the better. But it was tough and still is. I miss my best friend and sister who was always part of my life and joy, but I know I will see her again.

Two weeks later, September 11th happened, and the entire country was grieving everywhere we went and on TV, radio, etc., while we as a family were grieving for our loss. It was an extremely difficult time for our entire country, and grief was everywhere I turned. All I could do was cling to my Lord and Savior.

Because of Arlene's tremendous impact on so many children in the community, and of course her own, the line for her wake went outside and around the corner of the funeral home. There were huge articles about her in the newspaper, and her story was part of the local TV news. I had the honor and privilege again not only to help care for Arlene, but to give her eulogy. Senator George Maziarz also gave a eulogy, and her legacy lives on in so many people her short life touched. Arlene Wallak is now a special angel to her four boys, and is at peace in Heaven. I can't wait to be with her again.

Our faith and trust in God sustained my family and Arlene, as she walked through the valley of death and into Jesus's arms. When you go through something like that, there is no way to go through it alone, and you realize you make it through by God's incredible grace with a peace that surpasses all understanding.

I miss my sister more than you can imagine, and losing her affected me deep in my soul in ways I can't seem to put into words. Through that whole time Arlene was suffering, and since losing her, I felt closer to God than I had ever imagined. That was definitely a turning point for me in my faith. I had to look beyond our earth's shadows into what I could not see and trust in the Lord our Savior in order to go forward each and every day. That was one of those spiritual milestones of growth for me that I will never forget.

Losing my sister changed me in other ways too, as many of you know. I am more motivated to eat right and am passionate about teaching others to do the same to help prevent diseases like cancer, heart disease, and diabetes to name a few. I know I have a 50% risk of getting breast cancer myself, and that is part of what drives me every day. I did find a lump a few years ago, had a biopsy, and it was taken out with surgery. I thank God that it was negative.

What I'm driven by even more is knowing that Jesus died so I could have eternal life. It's living so that I can see Arlene again in Heaven, and the reality that I will live forever worshiping our Heavenly Father with her.

Today I care more about my eternal life and glorifying God in everything I do than anything else in the world. On top of that, God wants us to take care of our earthly bodies while we are here.

God created our mind, body, soul, and spirit for a reason. His divine principles tell us to take care of all four. I know I can't serve and glorify God on this earth and fulfill His purpose here in my life without my mind and body. I may not be here at all if I don't take care of my body.

Here is what I know. The answer to the "cure" that my sister asked me to be proactive about is right before our eyes—to PREVENT disease, to reverse disease, and to help spontaneous regression occur through a healthy lifestyle every day. We can't deny it: our lifestyle matters. If you can prevent disease and even reverse disease by eating right and exercising, why wouldn't you do that? I also know that God is sovereign, and He doesn't make mistakes.

We have a choice to LIVE every day, until we can't live anymore on this earth. And our mind-body connection is paramount. We must walk by faith, not by sight, and believe God is sovereign, because He is. But that doesn't mean we should just pray about everything and shouldn't make the right choices every day. We should pray about everything, yes, but we still have a responsibility to make the right choices and take care of our temples, the bodies God gave us. I knew if my sister lived, God didn't make a mistake, and I knew when God finally took her, that He didn't make a mistake. But in the meantime we did everything in our power for her to LIVE.

I realized over the years, that because of what I have gone through with both my parents and my sister, Arlene, helping others live has been my passion and my calling. And although I had an incident with my own health, which turned out okay, praise God, I know our life can change on a dime. None of us are guaranteed a tomorrow, but I know God is sovereign, and when we LIVE for HIM, and put our trust in HIM— He will make our paths straight, no matter what path that is. His will, not ours...

I am doing everything I can possibly do while I'm here in this little blip of a life to live out the promises I made to my sister. I learned so much from both my sister Arlene and my mom during those times in my life, and I know this—you CAN and SHOULD lean on God, and change your health.

You can prevent disease and even reverse disease. God made our bodies to heal themselves. And as my mom told me—at the ripe old age of 92, remember—until we leave this world, we should live life to its fullest. And that is what I intend to do.

Not a day or hour goes by when I don't think of my sister, mom, and dad. I miss them dearly. It's still difficult, but I know I will see them again and that gives me joy. Until then, I intend to LIVE life to the fullest, prevent disease, and help others LIVE to prevent disease. Because that, my friends, is the real "cure."

> *I know that absence with the body means present with the Lord. (2 Corinthians 5:6-8 and Philippians 1:21-23)*

As I mentioned earlier, I found a lump in my breast a few years back. And between the time that it was found, and the two months later when I had the surgery, it was gone. Nada. Tissue was sent in for testing, and nothing showed up cancerous.

Grace of God? Miracle? Absolutely I believe it was both. It was not my time, but I also took action. I was already eating right and exercising, but I of course continued praying, then tightened everything up, incorporating even more anti-cancer foods and therapies in my diet—and I'm still here!

My Dear Dad

My earthly father was older, and had had gray hair for as long as I could remember. He was twelve years older than my mom, and he was the first one to pass away in my immediate family, and that of course was tough. My dad, Robert, was a very loving Italian father who I was grateful to call "Dad." Not only was I named after him, but I think I was his favorite (just kidding). I was the youngest, and he was an accomplished artist by this time, and I spent a lot of time at his art shows with my mom. I was so proud of him.

Dad was a highly decorated World War II US Army Veteran in the 7th Division 106th Field Artillery, and he had all the medals and war stories to prove it. He loved his family, dogs, house parties, art, and music. He actually took us girls to see the Beatles in Toronto's Maple Leaf Gardens in 1965 and 1967 (OK look, I was young). In the line to get into the concert people thought he was famous because he always had a very distinguished look. So he told everyone that he was Cesar Romero and that he was in the show! Beatles fans said, "Who is Cesar Romero?" There was a definite generation gap!

Dad had been diagnosed with cancer in his late seventies, but he was generally feeling okay and seemed fine, with no chemo or radiation. I remember wondering at that time if the cancer was related to the power lines behind our house. Growing up, many people on our street had cancer. It may have been related to the power lines, and of course there was the Durez Corporation's chemical dump not far from us.

Life was going good until Dad had surgery on his spine when he was in his early eighties. I told Dad the risk of surgery at his age was too great, but he was determined that it would help his back pain. After surgery, unfortunately, he never walked again. We had been at my cousin's wedding the night before, and I have a picture of Dad and me slow dancing together the night before he became paralyzed forever. Little did I know what the next day would bring.

A few years later, a few days after Christmas, he would come down with pneumonia and pass away five days later on January 5th. We had a hospice room at the hospital for Dad, and he was most comfortable. As a nurse I was fully aware he was fading fast. I remember thinking that I did not want him to pass without us being with him. My sisters and my mom and I all slept over in the hospital. The night before Dad passed, I was sitting next to his bed reading Scripture to him and praying. My sisters and Mom had fallen asleep. I recall looking at the clock and noticing the exact time. I then fell asleep for literally five minutes, and when I woke up, Dad was gone—God took him. Just like that. Peaceful.

His tombstone, which he bought several years before he died, was engraved with words from his favorite song from Frank Sinatra: I did it my way. He sure did.

Family

So this chapter is about family, and I'm not only Italian, I'm also my mother's daughter! I have to admit, I love my house to be filled with family and friends who are like family! We talk, eat, laugh, eat, pray, eat, cry, eat, laugh, eat, work out, and eat some more.

To me, time with my family comes right after time with God. And I can't seem to get enough of either one. I start my day every morning thanking Him for all of the blessings in my life. I start with thanking and praying for my husband Jeff and our two daughters, who by the way are our gifts from God. I know my God-given job is to love my husband and train our children up the way they should go. God commands us to love one another, but I would do it anyway! Men are commanded to love their wives, and women are commanded to respect their husbands. Love and respect—those are two beautiful things.

We are also commanded to walk in the fruit of the Spirit.

> *But the fruit of the Spirit is love, joy, peace, patience, kindness, goodness, faithfulness, gentleness and self-control. (Galatians 5:22-23)*

Relationships and Marriage

I certainly am not an expert in this area, but there are a few things I know from God's Word. God does not want us to be alone.

> *The Lord God said "It is not good for man to be alone. I will make a helper suitable for Him." (Genesis 2:18)*

Research shows that the number one need of people is to feel loved and be forgiven. Relationships work best when we walk in the fruit of the Spirit. I was always one of those people who never liked being alone. I loved being in relationships and going on dates, and prayed early on as a teenager for a man who treated me right. Now back then I wasn't exactly praying for a godly Man, but I knew I should at least look for someone who really loved me and who I loved back. I was just going about my life as if I was in charge of who I would end up with. Boy, did I ever have a lot to learn.

But God – He knew what I needed and had it all in His plans from the start. I have been so blessed to have married a man of God. In fact on my first date with Jeff, he asked me if I wanted to pray with him! Wow! That was the first time any man had ever asked me to pray with him on a date. I thought right then and there that I wanted to marry this guy, and it was from that point on that I prayed I would.

My husband Jeff has been my rock over the years, but we have had our share of differences, trust me. We are opposites in so many ways and our marriage has had its up and downs like all marriages.

The one thing we had in common was our love for our Father God, and that was the most important thing. We always had the desire to follow God, but early in our dating years we hadn't really given our lives up and allowed Jesus to take over our life. But fortunately, God has been transforming both of us to be more like Him every day and we now have Him at the center of our marriage. No matter how bad things get, we know that Philippians 4:13 is true. We can do all things through Christ who strengthens us. We can't make it on our own.

Marriage is really two very imperfect people trying to have a perfect marriage, who don't want to give up on one another, and it is tough! Without God, many marriages wouldn't make it, and many don't. Satan will do whatever he can to break up marriages and families, and temptation is all around us. Some of the best marriages have had to endure the deepest pain, but in turn reach the highest level of joy as a result of working hard towards unity in the marriage.

We need to be in the Word daily, or things can derail very quickly. We are commanded to love and respect one another, and this is not easy as well, because we bring a lot of baggage and expectations from our past and what we witnessed in our own parents' marriage, plus we are selfish beings. Also, we are wired differently, perceptions come into play, and all of this causes us to see things differently creating misunderstanding. As my pastor says, "We allow lesser things to divide us, than allowing the Supreme Being to unite us." Love is the greatest commandment. Keep God at the center of your marriage and really fight with all your might for your marriage, it is worth it.

> *Though one may be overpowered, two can defend themselves. A cord of three strands is not quickly broken. (Ecclesiastes 4:12)*

> *Love the Lord your God with all your heart and with all your soul and with all your strength. This is the first and greatest commandment. And the second is like it: Love your neighbor as yourself. (Matthew 22:36)*

Marriage was God's idea, and it works out best when God is at the center of our marriages. It takes work, and it's not easy, but once it's clicking, it comes with a lot of pleasure and joy.

I find that people are always looking for the right person, but you need to *be* the right person for marriage to work out. It does take work and being selfless, no doubt about it. Pastor Gillis says, "Live a life that is worthy of the calling you receive." What we treasure is where we spend our time and energy, and that gets to the heart of what we think is worthy. We need to invest in our marriages. If you need professional help, get it. Make marriage your priority.

I never judge when people call it quits as none of us know what goes on in marriages and relationships. With that said since marriage is God's idea we should fight for it if at all possible. For couples so eager to call it quits and throw in the towel on your relationship because everything isn't 'perfect'...here is some food for thought. Lifelong commitment is not what most people think it is. It's not waking up every morning to make breakfast and eat together. It's not cuddling in bed until both of you fall asleep. It's not a clean home filled with laughter and love making everyday.

It's someone who steals all the covers, and snores, it's sometimes slammed doors and a few harsh words at times. It's stubbornly disagreeing and giving each other the silent treatment until your hearts heal, and then forgiveness. It's coming home to the same person everyday that you know loves and cares about you in spite of and because of who you are. It's laughing about the times you do something stupid. It's about dirty laundry and unmade beds. It's about helping each other with the hard work of life. It's about swallowing the nagging words instead of saying them out loud. It's about eating the easiest meal you can make and sitting down together at a late hour because you both had a crazy day. It's when you have an emotional breakdown and he/she holds you, and tells you everything is going to be OK. It's about still loving someone even though sometimes they make you absolutely insane. It's giving each other grace, lots of it. We all have our faults and all fall short of the glory of God. Loving someone isn't always easy, sometimes it's hard. But it is amazing and comforting and one of the best things you will ever experience.

Life isn't always about the highlight reel we post on social media where everything looks so perfect, and that's okay! Just know that with God all things are possible. Three strands aren't easily broken!

For where your treasure is, there your heart will be also.
(Luke 12:34)

Author Gary Thomas, in his book *The Sacred Marriage,* says:

> If happiness is our primary goal, we'll get a divorce as soon
> as happiness seems to wane. If receiving love is our primary
> goal, we'll dump our spouse as soon as they seem to be less
> attentive. But if we marry for the glory of God, to model
> His love and commitment to our children, and to reveal
> His witness to the world, divorce makes no sense.

Couples who've survived a potentially marriage-ending situation, such
as infidelity or a life-threatening disease, may continue to battle years
of built-up resentment, anger, or bitterness. So, what are some ways to
strengthen a floundering relationship, or even encourage a healthy one?
Thomas offers these practical tips:

- Focus on your spouse's strengths rather than their weaknesses.
- Encourage rather than criticize.
- Pray for your spouse and your marriage daily.

Learn and live what Christ teaches about relating to and loving others.

> *Love is patient, love is kind and is not jealous; love does not*
> *brag and is not arrogant, does not act unbecomingly; it does*
> *not seek its own, is not provoked, does not take into account a*
> *wrong suffered. (I Corinthians 13:4)*

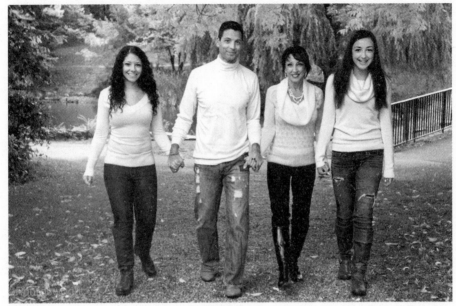

My family

Children

Our children are a gift from God, and I feel my highest calling is to be a loving and good parent and train my children up the way they should go. We are actually commanded by God to do just that. That takes time and patience and lots of understanding. Children need love, and as my mom always told me, "You can't love your children too much." She demonstrated that every day of her long life. I am so grateful for my two girls, Shanelle and Raquelle, and for my nephews who are like my own kids. I pray for them daily, several times a day, and know the power of prayer as a mother.

You know, there are many studies that show the effect of a strong support system with a loving environment on our mental and physical health, especially with babies' and the elderly's ability to thrive. We are commanded to love one another, be kind to one another, carry each other's burdens, and forgive one another the way Christ forgave us. And I'm sure you know that children will do what you do, not what you say! But it's also great to talk to your children, and even write a letter occasionally to tell them how much you love them or express things you want to say! I still have the letters Mom wrote me, and I will cherish them forever.

If you don't know what to say to them about God, but you're praying their eyes are open, or even if they are open, pray about it. Ask God to give you the words you need to say. You might write something like this:

Dear _____

If I were to be taken to Heaven today, there would be some important things I would want to say to you first. I have wisdom that you do not have, and that you have not tapped into. I think you are finding that life is not easy. Most people eventually get to a point where they throw their hands up in the air, or get down on their knees and say, "I can't do this alone!" Until that happens, many go through some heavy disappointments and years of soul searching. I was there.

First of all, no one will ever love you as deeply as Dad and I love you. We would go to the end of the world and back for you (and who else would do that?) A mother's love is also very special, as you have seen in my relationship with my own mother. Remember that I carried you for nine months inside of me, and we have a special bond unlike any other. You have only one Mom and Dad; be confident in knowing we want you to succeed more than anyone else on the planet does.

We may not be perfect parents, and you were not a perfect child at times, but God knew we were perfect for each other. No one is perfect except for the Lord. And I thank Him every day for you, and the wonderful blessing you are and have always been in my life.

I want to tell you how much I love you and how proud I am of you. I see all the greatness of the gifts and talents God has given you. You are smart, beautiful, funny, and have your whole future ahead of you.

Don't get discouraged that things aren't working out the way you hoped or as quickly as you hoped; they seldom do. God is working on things in your heart, and until you realize that you are not in control of your future, and that God is, you will be disappointed, upset, down in the dumps, and confused.

There are lessons He wants us to learn in life, and when you put your faith and trust in HIM and take your hands off the wheel, He will make your paths straight. It's normal to have doubts because you have never asked Him for help or have seen Him do His work in your life, and God will not force Himself on you! He gives us our own free will. But He asks us to walk by faith, and when we put our trust and hope in Him, He will give us the desires of our heart including hope and a great future!

The thing is, I can only help you with my prayers so much. And it's important to know that you can't really have a great future in this life, on your own will, good works, great looks, effort or greatness. God says that if you believe in Him and trust Him, you can't even imagine how great the future is that He has for you. I have seen this over and over in my life as well as in others.

I have seen God's hands all over my life! I have also seen miracles and the many supernatural things God has done that certainly were not a coincidence.

Life is tough, and the enemy will do everything he can to get you to believe his lies, to keep you doubting yourself so you stay away from God. There is so much joy and happiness waiting for you when you are ready to take that leap of faith. Ask, seek, knock, and the door will be open. Until then, God's face is turned away from us.

You should know that I am praying for you several times a day, and will continue to pray for you as long as I'm alive that you will have a long and wonderful future. I will also pray for you when I have eternal life, so my prayers will never end for you. Remember in the darkest of times, there is an answer. There is hope, and you can win the race when you just take that leap of faith and ask Jesus to take over your life.

I may be around for a long time, or I may go to Heaven tomorrow, but know that I love you. Whatever happens, I know I am going to Heaven. And I want to be sure that I will see you in Heaven, but I can't pray you into Heaven—you must take the step and leap of faith in God and ask Him to come into your life. I want the best for you and I am for you... and God is FOR us!

I love you,
Mom

Our character matters to God. And when we know God, it should be obvious in our parenting, in our marriage, at work and everywhere else. Yes, we are human, and Satan is always tempting us to mess up. But ask God to fill you with the Holy Spirit. Ask God to decrease you, and increase Him in your life. To take away anything that is not of Him. And when given the opportunity to shine, glorify God.

Friends like Family

Friends can be just like family, and I have certainly experienced that in my life. Jesus said in Mark 3:35, *Whoever does God's will is my brother and sister and mother.*

God made us to be connected with others, and isolation can work against us. Research has shown how critical it is for us to have a strong support system and be connected to one another, to support each other's goals and help one another through the challenges. Having that support system is important to our health, and also to living out the abundant life that God desires for us.

The research has also shown that we become most like the closest five people we hang out with. In a study published in the *New England Journal of Medicine*, researchers found that one of the strongest associations in the spread of obesity are the people you hang out with. Subjects who had a friend who was obese had a 57% chance of also being obese. If the two people considered themselves close friends, the figure shot up to 71%.

The good news is, there is a vast amount of research that shows that healthy habits are contagious. If you spend time with people who exercise and eat right, you are more likely to exercise and eat right. I certainly have seen that in my own life.

I love that my friends and I encourage one another to eat healthy and exercise. It's not even a verbal encouragement, it's just something we are all interested in, and therefore it's what we do when we are together. I can't imagine saying to one of my friends, "Let's go out and have a piece of cake and coffee!" It's just not something I would even think nowadays, nor would they. We go out to healthy places to eat and have healthy food! And we talk about our workouts, classes, and schedules to fit it all in. We encourage one another by our lifestyles.

Of course the fact that we all love God brings us together in even a greater way, to encourage one other and pray for one another. I don't know what I would have done without my friends when my mom was transitioning to heaven. Not only did I see bags of food dropped off in my kitchen each time I came out of Mom's room, but the text messages, phone calls, prayers, and support I received are something I will never ever forget.

I am blessed with a lot of wonderful friends who have supported me over the years, and I appreciate them all. But I have only a few very close friends who have been with me through thick and thin over the years, who I let into my struggles and joys, and who have stood by me in the good times and bad. These friends are like sisters to me, and I cherish those relationships more than I can say. Value, serve, and love those friends who are there for you and be there for them. And as my mom said, "Hang on to your good friends. They are as precious as diamonds." I intend to.

Attacks and Forgiveness

With family, we need the most patience and understanding. But unfortunately within the family, sometimes you'll find family members are most critical of one another. The more important the relationship, the deeper the pain can be, but the greater the joy, as family is most important. You may even see each other at your worst when your guard is down, as we are all human. And the family may be the most difficult place to be a witness for God. You may be expected to be perfect because you are following Christ, and others may not realize or admit that none of us are perfect. All of us fall short of the glory of God. Pastor Jerry Gillis says that "sometimes we are too busy watching and complaining instead of watching and praying." Instead of complaining about what's wrong with the world and the people in it, we should just continue to watch what's happening but pray for His will to be done.

Remember that Christ's family rejected and ridiculed Him? Jesus knows what you face by trying to be a witness for Him in your family. Stay true to your faith in spite of the attacks.

The more effective you are as a follower of Christ, the greater your attacks from the enemy. There are some that will accuse you of the most ridiculous things and may convince others they are sincere and telling the truth. Stand firm in God's truth, because you know He sees your heart and the real truth. God permits Satan to work in our world, but God is still in control. Jesus has power over Satan because He is God, and one day Satan will be bound forever (Revelation 20:10).

God's Word is clear about forgiveness. We are to forgive others as God forgave us. God teaches us about revenge and loving our enemies in Matthew 5:38-48. When we are wronged, our first reaction is to get even. Instead, God says we should be good to those who have wronged us! Our desire should not be to keep score and build up hatred.

We need to love and forgive, and this is not of the natural world, but with God it can happen supernaturally. Only God can give us the strength to love and forgive. Scripture tells us instead of building up a wall, or vengeance, to pray for those who hurt you. Many times people are upset with themselves, and they deflect on you. Know that you don't need to take that on. Just pray for them, and forgive them.

God tells us to make peace with our brothers and sisters, and we certainly should attempt to do that with prayer, realizing that we all fall short of the Glory of God.

God says,

Blessed are the pure at heart for they will see God. (Matthew 5:8)

Blessed are the peacemakers for they will be called Sons of God. (Matthew 5:9)

Blessed are those who are persecuted because of righteousness, for theirs is the Kingdom of Heaven. (Matthew 5:10)

God teaches about anger and says:

But I tell you, anyone who is angry with his brother will be subject to judgment. (Matthew 5:22)

If you have tried to make peace with those who hurt you or you have hurt, lay your burdens down at the feet of Jesus. And never stop praying for them and for restoration of the relationship. Satan loves to get in between marriages, family members, and friends. But of course, God can prevent and restore broken relationships, again supernaturally.

Until restoration takes place, we don't need to choose to be around those friends or family who continually hurt or persecute us. You can exercise and eat right all day long, but if you are constantly in a hurtful relationship, it can eventually be toxic to your mental and physical health. Continue to pray, and do something about your situation if you can. Be productive. Journaling or expressing yourself in writing is always good. Either write something worth reading, or do something worth writing that can help others.

You may not forget what someone said or has done, but always forgive as we were forgiven. Keep the faith, always love, always forgive, and don't be afraid to say you are sorry even if you don't believe you did anything wrong. I always think, "What would my Mom do?" because she was a peacemaker, and she loved with all her heart. But the bottom line is, of course, WWJD?

Bearing with one another and, if one has a complaint against another, forgiving each other; as the Lord has forgiven you, so you also must forgive. (Colossians 3:13)

The first to apologize is the bravest, the first to forgive is the strongest, the first to forget is the happiest. And the fact of the matter is our life can change on a dime. Our life can be gone in an instant without out any warnings. So drop the drama and love one another before it's too late.
—Author Unknown

God opposes the proud, but gives grace to the humble. (James 4:6)

Some good words to live by:

Watch your thoughts, for they become words.
Watch your words, for they become actions.
Watch your actions, as they become habits.
Watch your habits, for they become character.
Watch your character, for they become your destiny.

—Author unknown

If possible, so far as it depends on you, be at peace with all men. (Romans 12:18)

Be kind to one another, tenderhearted, forgiving one another as God and Christ forgave you. (Ephesians 4:32)

Health Advocate

When it comes to health care, fight for your family and be your own health advocate.

By definition, an advocate is one who argues or pleads another's cause. You have to be your own health advocate when you are eating the right foods and exercising, but also deciding to be proactive about preventing disease and asking questions. My mom grew up in an era where she never questioned the doctors or health care professionals. Today, that has changed. My mom, sister, and dad couldn't be their own health advocates toward the last years of their lives, and I believe God gave that job to me for them, and I am so forever grateful. Whenever a health concern arises, I am with my family every step of the way asking questions, and if I'm the patient, I ask my own questions, and I put all of my faith in Christ.

The list can go on and on but the bottom line is, if you're going to fight to stay fit and healthy in the gym, you better do the same thing outside the gym in the doctor's office or hospital. Don't be afraid to ask questions, and make sure you're satisfied with the answers you get before moving on. And most important, trust in God alone, and listen when God speaks to you. When you know something is wrong, don't take modern medicine as the gospel. God's Word is the Gospel and He is in control. God will do His work in us and in our situation no matter what it may be. He is holy, all-mighty, righteous, pure, all-knowing, all-powerful, and all-wise.

Trust in the Lord with all your heart and lean not on your own understanding; in all your ways acknowledge Him, and He will make your paths straight. (Proverbs 3:5-6)

And we know that in all things God works for the good of those who love Him, who have been called according to His purpose. (Romans 8:28)

All in all… whether or not you have that strong family network and support system, you can rest assured that God loves you!

7 Truths About Family to Help You On Your Journey:

1. Be humble, sympathetic, patient and kind. Walk in the fruit of the spirit with your family and others (1 Peter 3:8-9). Build up and encourage one another. Be kind, compassionate and forgiving (Ephesians 4:29). Remember serving others shows glory to God (Colossians 3:23).
2. Practice love and respect in your marriage.
3. Remember children are a gift from God. Tell them you love them daily. Listen to your children with intent, and train them up the way they should go. Children need our guidance and our time.
4. Honor your mother and father (Exodus 20:12). Call your mother and/or father often and tell them you love them.
5. Maintain self-control at all times. (Galatians 5:22-23)
6. Lay your burdens down. Give it all to God. Seek Him first in all that you do and He will direct your paths.
7. Ask the God of the universe to take up residence in your heart. Offer yourself as a living sacrifice and ask God to use you for His glory in all arenas of your life, and be a light to others. (Romans 12)

Whatever the circumstance or trials, remember God will be glorified through them. (Ephesians 3:20-21)

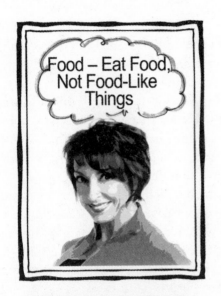

Food – Eat Food, Not Food-Like Things

TRUTH THREE

Food – Eat Food, Not Food-Like Things

W E HAVE AN astronomical obesity epidemic going on, but many who are obese are starving at the cellular level! We have obese children who will become obese adults, resulting in even more people with diseases associated with obesity, such as heart disease, diabetes, and cancer. We need to break the chain, and change and improve our health, and the good news is, we have the "technology" to do it! It's called food, the food of the earth that God created!

Here's the thing: God cares more about the condition of our heart than the condition of our bodies, but we need to take care of the body God gave us! Our "mobile homes," our "temporary earth suits," as I like to call them.

Health care should not be about medication, the FDA, the RDA, or anything else. It's really about what I do every day in making people well, preventing and reversing disease through their lifestyle habits, and bio-individuality.

As a registered nurse for many years, I took care of sick people. I decided I wanted to switch gears and do what I call "preventative nursing," to help people prevent disease and be healthy. I realized early on in talking with my patients and researching their diseases, that many of them could have prevented disease and stayed out of the hospital simply by changing their lifestyle habits. I also realized that we pay more for our health care than any other country, but we don't have better health to show for it.

During those early years, I spent most of my health and fitness career focusing on exercise, the scale, and what size jeans I wore. I thought I had the right motivation, but that was far from the truth. What I weighed would either make or break my day. My self-worth revolved around the scale. If I was even a couple of pounds up, I would feel bad about myself, and somehow that scale became the measuring stick for everything.

I was in 11th grade and sixteen years old when I convinced my mom to let me join European Health Club. Most of my friends didn't even know what a health club was. I thought that exercising would be the answer to feeling better, looking better, being happy, and staying lean. At least that's what Cher portrayed on the commercials.

So I exercised every chance I got, lost a little weight, then started eating anything I wanted, gaining it all back. I would gain and lose five to ten pounds several times over, and when you are 5'2" that's a whole size up or down. Of course I was still thin in most people's eyes at sizes 4 to 8, but it was a constant struggle with myself to stay thin.

It was then that I first realized that you can't "out-exercise" a bad diet. So I started "dieting." I lived mostly on salads but would still have bouts of bingeing on junk food, mainly sweets, which I craved more than real food. I could eat cookie dough no problem, and although this was not the norm for me, dieting was—and I tried every diet in the book! The protein diet, the low-carb diet, the low-calorie diet, the low-fat diet, the no-fat diet, and the list went on and on. None of them actually worked, and all of them wreaked havoc on my health and metabolism. I was struggling to find the key to eat what I wanted and not get fat. No one knew of this struggle, not even my close friends.

I believe my mom could see my heart, however, as moms know you like no other. When I wanted to eat dessert as soon as I walked in the house, she would just gently and lovingly guide me by saying, "Don't ruin your appetite and eat that now, honey. Wait for dinner." Truly, I would rather have desserts than her wonderful dinner! Most of the time I listened to Mom, and when I didn't, I would always come to the conclusion that she was right.

Exercising every chance you get and eating mostly salads will make you lose weight eventually. But it's not the right way, and your body will crave the nutrients it desperately needs.

Later on in my late teens, through early twenties, I still had a preoccupation with food and dieting. I would binge and starve myself and go on every diet out there in an effort to be thin. At that time, I still didn't realize that being thin didn't obviously equate to being healthy. I exercised like crazy, skipped meals, and was not healthy by any stretch of the imagination. I focused on calories in and calories out but never changed the shape of my body, cut cravings, felt good, or was healthy. I was a sugar addict, and I knew it!

I felt I was a failure because I couldn't seem to get a handle on this "diet thing" and kick the sugar. Looking back, I don't exactly know where my own preoccupation with dieting came from, as my mom always built me up and made me feel beautiful. I know she and God loved me, but somehow that didn't seem like enough. But did I really know God? The answer was no, not yet.

I loved taking fitness classes at European Health Club, and this was when group classes had just started to be a part of the fitness scene. This is when I met my best and longtime friend Valerie. One day one of the Fitness Managers asked me if I wanted to teach classes. I was shocked! Me? Teach?

I didn't feel good enough, thin enough, or fit enough to be a fitness instructor! But people at the gym encouraged me. I thought, they must think I can do it, and I love taking classes, so why not? Soon after I was teaching and that made me feel a little better about myself, as people starting giving me feedback that they enjoyed my motivation and energy. Little did they know I was not as healthy and fit as I looked. I was still a sugar addict.

As a result of being "on stage," that also began a period where I felt tremendous pressure to "look and act the part" of an instructor. How could I let them know I'd rather eat chocolate-chip cookies than salads if I'm a fitness instructor? As time went on, I did start eating better, but I was still a sugar-holic and it was a slippery slope when I had any sugar at all!

I once again lost weight, a lot of weight, from dieting and exercising, but I was far from healthy, and of course eventually I started gaining it all back and then some.

I started being interested in health in general, and bought a juicer at that time, then started juicing carrots like they were going out of style. Back then juicing was not even part of the English vocabulary like it is today. I would literally juice five pounds of carrots at one time and drink the whole thing. My hair started to fall out from too much Vitamin A, and I was losing muscle tone from not enough protein. I started adding in protein but again really didn't know what I was doing, and my weight continued to fluctuate as I searched for that magic bullet. At one time, I was thirty pounds heavier than I am today. And it was not muscle. Of course I yo-yoed down again with some other crazy diet, and the madness continued.

Look, I'm Italian, and I love to eat!! My mom's house was the dessert capital of the world. We had pasta and bread, pasta and potatoes, bread and more pasta and always dessert to finish it off. As I said, I was 30 pounds heavier than I am today, and it was not muscle! Then, one of those days, I woke up and said, 'today is the day!' I planned on wiping the slate clean and was going to start eating healthy and losing weight. Lo and behold, I didn't do it. In fact, I failed and had a hot fudge sundae to start my day! Of course I felt bad about that, felt out of control, and said tomorrow I am going to start all over so I might as well have another—and then I had another! Three ice cream sundaes in one day!

Now, they were tiny and one scoop of ice cream each, but it doesn't matter! That was one of my lowest points, when I had no self-control with food, and I was continually trying to sabotage myself!

But God knew the desire of my heart to honor and glorify Him with my body, and eventually with God I turned it around. Not only did I turn it around, but I have now spent the last thirty-five-plus years helping to inspire others who also were in a rut or just needed a tune-up. The good news is we can do something about getting out of that rut—we can break the chain no matter what our upbringing was or what our own history is, and we should!

I graduated from nursing school in 1982 and I also became certified to teach classes that same year in the first-ever Fitness Certification in New York City. It was at that time that I began learning more about body composition, health and nutrition in the practical sense of the word rather than just what I learned in nursing about the science of "nutrition." You see, what I learned about in school was what many health care practitioners and doctors learned in school: the old food pyramid, which suggested we eat six to eleven servings of grains per day, and calories in, and calories out. No wonder we had an obesity problem!

In the 90s, I became friends with a girl who was taking my classes, who I will call Mary. She was a regular in my classes, and I thought she was a picture of health. She was thin, and pretty, and energetic. I eventually asked her to start teaching my classes for me as I branched out. I plugged her into the different locations I taught at, and she taught my signature program called "Peak Performance," which later turned into "Raw Energy."

I finally started to get a handle on the whole eating right thing, but it was around that time that I began to see Mary lose more and more weight as time went on. I began to get very concerned that she was dieting like I had done in the past, but it was obvious it was more extreme. It's funny how when you've experienced something yourself, you have a strong sense of intuition when someone else is doing the same thing.

People would comment to Mary how thin she was getting, and her face would light up. I remember asking her once what she ate that day, and she told me she had one piece of bread, all day! I thought to myself—one piece of bread? How does she survive on that? One day when we were hanging out, I happened to notice that there was literally nothing in Mary's refrigerator but a bottle of water! That same week she jumped on the scale at the club in front of me, and the scale said ninety pounds. She had been 125 just months earlier. I knew then something was terribly wrong with Mary, and I felt compelled to tell someone in an effort to help her, but who? I really didn't know her family that well.

At that time I was working as a nurse and also the aerobic director at my gym. I decided to call Mary's mom and expressed my concern that she was losing so much weight so fast. Her mom didn't seem that alarmed, or maybe she just wasn't letting on to me that she was. I told her mom that I thought Mary should see a doctor to make sure she was okay, and that I decided I would take Mary off the teaching schedule for a bit. I took Mary off the schedule the very next week without giving her a reason; however, I believe she knew the exact reason why. Little did I know that within one month of my taking Mary off the schedule, without any warning, Mary died of what I was told was a cardiac arrest at the "ripe old" age of twenty-five. My friend died! I was devastated. Did she starve herself to death? I never did find out, as everything was hush-hush.

One thing was for sure: I didn't want what happened to Mary to happen to anyone else. Losing Mary affected me profoundly. It was then that my struggle and preoccupation with the scale began to diminish, and my faith in God grew deeper. After years of struggling to seek happiness, acceptance, and peace as a teenager, the Lord began to speak into my spirit: *I don't care what the scale says. I created you, I love you,* and *I care for every part of you.* And the transformation of my mind, body, soul, and spirit began. I finally had a breakthrough in an area of struggle where I felt I had no hope, and that, of course, was something only God could do.

You see, we really aren't healthy unless we are healthy in our mind, body, soul, and spirit. It's all integrated. Our faith, family, food, fitness, sleep, stress, and health all matter. But the most important thing about us is what we think about God.

It was also after Mary died that my career started going in a different direction, and I found what I believe is God's purpose in my life today: helping people get healthy and fit spiritually as well as physically. I now believe this is my calling.

I started looking at food as something God gave us to heal and fuel our bodies. Not merely for taste, or to satisfy cravings, to fill an emotion, or to fill boredom, but actually to help us live. When the situation with my sister followed, her journey sealed the deal for me in terms of convincing me that real food was medicine, and junk food was poison.

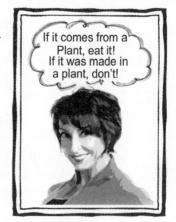

The science of eating healthy and staying lean and mean is not rocket science, but there is a science to it, which I will present in this chapter. In a nutshell, here are three Raw Truths:

1) We need to eat nutrient-dense foods, which are the foods of the earth that God has created, including lots of vegetables, and exercise at least 30 minutes per day or more every day to help us live longer, feel better, and prevent disease.
2) The God that created the body can heal the body and has given us the foods of the earth just for that reason!
3) It's really fairly simple. If it comes from a plant, eat it. If it was made in a plant, don't eat it!

If you want to stay out of the doctor's office and feel great, you need to exercise and eat right. So why don't you? You say you don't have time? Listen, no one has time—you simply make time because it's that important to the quality of your life, your level of fitness, your body composition, and your mental and physical health.

Our health care system says, "Just take this medication, but don't worry about changing your diet." There is something seriously wrong with that system when I hear from my patients that their doctors or health practitioners will prescribe medication for diabetes, high cholesterol, or high blood pressure, but not talk to them about their diet. Just take your medication and eat what you want? That's not health care, it's sick care!

First of all, let's get this clear: I can give you all the best cutting-edge health, nutrition, and fitness information in the world but without God nothing is possible! We need God to transform us in His image. And, if we seek God first, He will make our paths straight (health, fitness, weight loss, finances, marriage, children, Godliness) and that list goes on and on.

> *Trust in the Lord with all your heart and lean not on your own understanding; in all your ways acknowledge Him, and He will make your paths straight. (Proverbs 3:5-6)*

> *And we know that in all things God works for the good of those who love Him, who have been called according to His purpose. (Romans 8:28)*

We need self-control to get on, and stay on, the right track. My pastor said it this way: "Self-control can be defined as Spirit-given strength to be mastered by nothing but God."

We all need that strength, as there are temptations all around us, like overindulging in food or anything else. We need to be deliberate about our choices and keep our eyes on Christ our Savior. We need to persevere through our trials. Perseverance can be defined as faith-filled endurance to follow Jesus all the way home—I love that. Sign me up!

The Raw Truth Recharge is so much more than losing weight, staying lean, and getting in shape. It's a transformation of mind, body, soul, and spirit. One thing I know for sure is that God wants us to take care of our temples where the Holy Spirit dwells so we can glorify Him!

For one thing, we need to have energy to go out and do God's work. If we are sick, thick, and tired every day we won't have the energy to get up out of bed, let alone make a difference in the lives of the people around us. How do I know this? Because I was sick and thick and tired myself back then. I craved sugar and junk food and thought I could out-exercise my bad diet by teaching twenty-five classes a week. I found out that didn't work, and boy, did I have a lot to learn!

Yesterday, You Said Tomorrow

It's now or never, my friends! Get your head and heart in the game and transform your life and health, forever.

Remember that people who don't eat right and take care of their bodies now will have to live with the consequences later. Be it more weight and less energy now or disease later. And our choices matter—mentally, physically, emotionally, and spiritually.

God's Word is clear:

> *Do you not know that your body is a temple of the Holy Spirit, who is in you, whom you have received from God? You are not your own; you were bought at a price. Therefore honor God with your body. (1 Cor. 6:19-20)*

Bio-individuality

With healthy eating, working out, and detoxing, one size does not fit all. And in my private practice I am able to prescribe protocols according to individual needs in a prescription called **bio-individuality**. The concept of bio-individuality is that each of us has unique food, nutrition, and lifestyle needs. One person's body functions better with a plant-based diet, where another person's body functions better by including some animal products. Working on the principle of bio-individuality, it's important for health practitioners to evaluate our patients' needs, then suggest positive changes that are based on their unique needs, health history, medications, lifestyle, preferences, and ancestral background.

And by the way, your genes (and jeans) are not your fate. Just because your family is unhealthy or obese doesn't mean you have to be! And just because you were obese growing up, or you craved junk food as a teenager, doesn't mean you need to as an adult. Break the chain with a detox and start craving what your body needs. More on detox in the next chapter!

Think about the fact that diseases are being prevented, and even start to reverse themselves, when we start eating right and exercising. And the results are immediate, the moment you change your diet. Start eating right and exercising today and you will start being healthier today! How could you not want to change your life and prevent or reverse disease? The choice is yours! Why would you not want to make that choice?

I have heard people say to me that they are going to smoke or eat the foods that kill them as much as they want, and if they die from that, then at least they will die happy! Really? You don't care that you wake up sick and thick and tired every day? And you don't care that the people who love you and want you to live will be left behind because of your bad habits? I just don't understand.

Over the past thirty-plus years, I have run into countless people who think they are eating right because they are following the food recommendations made by our government and the commercials on TV. The standard American diet is killing us, and so are the Canadian and worldwide recommendations for that matter!

Our health care system is really sick care! Do you know that our government has been subsidized to push certain foods on us? And our government will approve something like aspartame, which crosses the blood brain barrier and causes things like tinnitus (ringing in the ears) and other major health problems, but they have trouble approving things made from a plant, like Stevia for instance?

What better day than today to start eating better and taking care of the "mobile home," our "earth suits," that God gave us. Start by renewing your mind and saying, "I am able" with God. "I am able to do whatever I need to do thru Christ who strengthens me."

Look away from those things that distract us. Change your focus from food to God and pray for strength and self-control. Put a Post-it on your refrigerator that says, "We can do this together, I am with you and for you. – Love God." And know you are worth it!

The Raw Truth Recharge is based on the low glycemic index, nutrient-dense foods of the earth that God created. The objectives are to fuel your body with the foods it needs to grow, prevent disease, reverse disease, and heal. The Raw Truth Recharge will help you to increase or maintain muscle mass, and decrease body fat through your dietary habits and workout, and to avoid the foods that flip on the metabolic switch that signals your body to store fat. Muscle dictates metabolism, which is why building and maintaining muscle is so important.

Muscle Dictates Metabolism

Here's the Raw Truth: you can build muscle two ways—through training and working out, and through what you eat. Calorie-restrictive diets sabotage us completely and decrease our metabolism about 15% due to the restriction in calories. The worst thing you can do is slow down your metabolism when you are trying to lose weight, burn fat, and increase muscle mass. When you drastically reduce your calories, your body doesn't know the difference between being stuck in the wilderness without any food or being in your kitchen with cupboards full of food and water, and just not eating or drinking on purpose! God made our body so that it protects us when we are stuck in the wilderness or in trouble, by slowing down our metabolism and hanging onto fat. When we skip meals or drastically reduce our calorie intake, that is exactly what happens.

Calories do matter somewhat. But if fitness was just about calories in and calories out, then everyone who is killing themselves in the gym would be lean and mean. I never cared about calories, and I don't count them at all now, because I'm active, and what I eat is nutrient-dense. I *need* calories to do what I do each day, and so do you!

And what about counting points? If you tell me you can have processed food or junk food because it only has 1 or 2 points, that doesn't make sense! The Raw Truth, again, is that eating healthy is not counting calories, counting points, weighing, measuring, or eliminating whole food groups. It's learning day-by-day, week-by-week how to change your eating habits and make better choices. It's about how to choose foods that don't flip on the metabolic switch to store fat. It's about eating to fuel our bodies and heal our bodies. God created those foods to do just that!

The Raw Truth Recharge is not a diet because diets don't work. It's a lifestyle program based on behavior modification, education, and motivation. It's an immunity-boosting, body-shaping, healthy living, low glycemic protocol that fuels our body. It's about eating whole, nutrient-dense foods of the earth that God created (good carbs, lean protein, veggies and a little fruit).

Understanding The Glycemic Index and Load

The Glycemic Index

You've seen me mention the glycemic index, so let me explain what that means since it's so important to our health.

The Glycemic Index (GI) is a measure to which a carbohydrate is likely to raise your blood sugar (glucose) levels. The scale is 0 to 100 with 0 being low and 100 being high. The GI compares equal quantities of carbohydrates and provides a measure of carbohydrate quality *but not quantity*. So the drawback with GI ratings is that they are not based on commonly consumed portion sizes of foods.

Studies have linked a high glycemic diet to insulin-resistant Type 2 diabetes, obesity, high cholesterol, increased risk of cardiovascular disease, and some cancers. If that doesn't motivate you, maybe this will. Studies have linked weight loss, improved blood sugar, lower triglycerides, cholesterol, and fat loss to a low-glycemic system.

Some of you think because you are avoiding sugar you are eating low-glycemic, but it's not just about the sugar you add to your foods or eat. The sweetness of a food doesn't necessarily correlate with the glycemic index. Sweet potatoes have a much lower glycemic index than white potatoes. It's not about the foods you eat; it's about the impact that those foods have on blood sugar, which then causes your body to gain weight.

Although carrots have a higher glycemic index, the amount ingested would be equivalent to one and half pounds of carrots consumed—far more, of course, than people normally eat as a snack or part of a meal. The GI rating often overstates or understates a relatively small carbohydrate content in a food item like a carrot. Therefore, I recommend using the Glycemic Load (GL) index with calculations also based upon realistic portions. GL ranks food according to the effects of actual carbohydrate content in a standard serving size of food.

GI value ranges from 1-100:

- Low is 1-55
- Medium is 56-69
- High is 70-100

Glycemic Load index

In 1997, Harvard University scientists introduced the concept of Glycemic Load (GL). This measure gives a more accurate reflection of the blood sugar effects of a standard food portion. To simplify it, the GL of a typical serving of food is the amount of available carbohydrates in that serving and the glycemic index of that food.

The higher the GL of a food, the greater the expected rise in blood glucose, and the greater the adverse insulin effects of the food. Foods with a GL of 10 or below would be presumed to be less detrimental to health, while those with a GL of 20 and above would have more detrimental effects. Long-term consumption of foods with a high glycemic load appears to be linked to a greater risk of obesity, diabetes, and inflammation.

There are several factors that affect whether a food will spike your blood sugar:

- The number one factor is how much fiber a food contains or doesn't contain. Fiber lowers the glycemic index of foods, which is why it's important to eat foods with at least 5 grams of fiber.
- The extent of processing of the food affects the GI. The more processed it is the higher the glycemic index. Sprouted bread is better than processed bread.
- The extent of cooking affects the GI. The more you cook foods, even vegetables, the higher the glycemic index.
- Acid content affects the GI.
- The type of starch or sugar a food contains affects the GI naturally.

Some foods are low in the glycemic index (e.g., sugar-free) but high in bad fat, which will be just as detrimental to your success as drastically reducing your caloric intake or GI. So just because something is low in the glycemic index does not mean it's healthy.

Without getting too technical, different types of carbohydrates are processed differently in the body and consequently affect your blood sugar differently. There are simple carbs and complex carbs. Simple carbs include table sugar, which you want to stay away from, while complex carbohydrates are broken down by the body more slowly. All unprocessed fruits and veggies, grains, beans, and nuts contain both digestible and non-digestible carbs.

Digestible carbohydrates can be used by the body for fuel; indigestible carbs can't be used in the body.

When reading a label, you will see that carbohydrates are broken down as follows: sugar, dietary fiber, sugar alcohols, and other carbohydrates. You may see "net carbs" listed on a label, as many companies are starting to share that information so we don't have to do the math. That number of net carbs tells how much the carbohydrates you are eating will impact your blood sugar levels—again, the glycemic index. You should aim for single digits and nutrient-dense ingredients.

Net Carbs = Carbohydrates – fiber – sugar alcohol (look for single digits)
Glycemic load + GI + amount of carb (look for less than 10)

So why is this so important? The bottom line: if you regularly consume a high glycemic index diet, you have a higher chance of developing a number of serious health problems including insulin-resistant diabetes, obesity, cancer, and cardiovascular disease. A low-glycemic diet helps you keep your weight down while lowering cholesterol, increasing energy, stabilizing your blood sugar, and promoting overall mental and physical health. There are many other side effects of a high-glycemic diet, like lethargy and irritability, which most people don't even consider.

There's more. Did you know that brown bananas have a higher glycemic index than yellow-green bananas? Did you know that brown rice, although it has more vitamins and minerals than white, has a glycemic index almost on par with white rice and bread? And a white baked potato does the same thing in your body as a piece of dessert? And we wonder why people aren't losing weight eating what they think is healthy food!

What Low GI Eating Can Do:

- Improve your energy level
- Increase weight loss
- Improve body composition (more muscle less fat)
- Improve your health
- Help cut the cravings and hunger
- Stop the metabolic switch that signals your body to store fat as fuel
- Reduce your risk of a heart attack by 4 to 11%
- Decrease your risk for diabetes

Here are a couple more general food guidelines.

- Foods that rob your energy and make you fat include white bread, rice, flour and sugar, pop, potatoes, sweets, processed food, and toxins.
- Foods that fuel your body **include** water, veggies, fruits, whole grain, sprouted grain, beans, legumes and good sources of protein, nuts and good fats, and foods of the earth.

THE MACRONUTRIENTS

Protein and Fat and Carbohydrates

Macronutrients are nutrients that provide calories or energy. Nutrients are substances needed for growth, metabolism, and for other body functions. Since "macro" means large, macronutrients are nutrients needed in large amounts. There are three macronutrients: Proteins, Fats and Carbohydrates. We are going to look at all three and how essential they are to our health.

PROTEIN

"Whaddya mean you don't eat no meat? That's ok! That's ok! I make lamb!"

Do you remember that part in the movie, *My Big Fat Greek Wedding*? Well, that was life at my dear mother's house every day in so many ways!

I loved my mom more than life itself, but each and every day on top of dessert, she would offer me meatballs, steak, pork chops, etc. Even after I hadn't eaten that stuff in some thirty years, she was always amazed and concerned that I didn't eat meat!

Mom was constantly asking me, "Where do you get your protein from?" and "Why don't the girls drink milk? They need it to grow!" Or say things like, "You look too thin—you're not eating!" and "I like you more puffy!" So then I'd have to go into my loving dissertation again about how I eat all day long, what I ate today, and that I get my protein from other (better) sources like plants, lentils, nuts, quinoa, beans, hemp bagels, sprouted grain bread, eggs, non-GMO tofu, plants, fish, etc. Mom didn't quite understand the whole no milk, no meat thing, but hopefully you will. You don't need to eat meat to get your protein. In fact, Non-GMO Soybean Sprouts contain 54% protein, Soybean Curds (Tofu) 43%, Spirulina (plant algae) 60%, Spinach 49%, Kale and Broccoli 45%, Bussels Sprouts 44%, Turnip Greens and Collards 43%, and the list goes on and on.

A plant based-diet is an anti-cancer diet and much healthier for you all the way around. You do need to make sure you are getting enough Vitamin B12 if you are a Vegetarian, since all Vitamin B12 comes from animal sources. Take a good supplement and eat foods containing Vitamin B12 like cereals and Tofu. Plants trump meat in terms of the amount of protein they have, and you know how much better plants are for you! I haven't eaten beef in more than thirty years, and I know my body is healthier because of it.

Protein's role in your body is very important, from building tissues to forming vital antibodies, hormones, and enzymes. Getting a regular supply of protein is essential because your body doesn't store it for future use. It also helps you lose weight because it's slowly digested, which makes you feel full, and it takes more calories to digest proteins than carbs.

Animal protein promotes the growth of cancer. In his book *The China Study*, author T. Colin Campbell, PhD., talks about growing up on a dairy farm, where he regularly enjoyed a wholesome glass of milk. He doesn't any more. In multiple, peer-reviewed animal studies, researchers discovered that milk and dairy could actually turn the growth of cancer cells on and off by raising and lowering doses of casein, the main protein found in cow's milk.

Plants are powerful. Dr. Campbell's study showed that "People who ate the most animal-based foods got the most chronic disease. People who ate the most plant-based foods were the healthiest."

Caldwell B. Esselstyn Jr. M.D., a physician and researcher who practiced at The Cleveland Clinic, treated thousands of patients with established coronary disease with a whole foods, plant-based diet. Not only did the intervention of a plant-based diet stop the progression of the disease, but also 70 percent of the patients saw an opening of their clogged arteries.

And it's not just cancer and heart disease that respond to a whole foods, plant-based diet. It may also help protect you from diabetes, obesity, autoimmune diseases, bone, kidney, eye, and brain diseases.

Many people nowadays have decided to go vegetarian. But what does that mean exactly?

Types of Vegetarians

- Vegans don't eat any animal products whatsoever (no meat, cheese, dairy, fish, etc.). They also do not consume eggs and dairy. True vegans also do not use honey or beeswax, gelatin, or any other animal by-product or ingredients.
- Pescatarians/Pescetarians: While technically not a type of vegetarian, these individuals do restrict their meat consumption to fish and seafood only. Pescatarians do not consume red meat, white meat, or fowl. They are considered "semi-vegetarians."
- Pollotarians: Much like the pescatarian, these "semi-vegetarians" restrict their meat consumption to poultry and fowl only. Pollotarians do not consume red meat or fish and seafood.
- Flexitarians: These folks do their best to limit meat intake as much as possible, and they have an almost entirely plant-based diet. This is not technically considered a "vegetarian" diet, but these people sometimes refer to themselves as vegetarians.
- Lacto-Vegetarians: Lacto-vegetarians do not eat red or white meat, fish, fowl, or eggs. However, lacto-vegetarians do consume dairy products such as cheese, milk, and yogurt.

- Ovo-Vegetarian: Ovo-vegetarians do not eat red or white meat, fish, fowl, or dairy products. However, ovo-vegetarians do consume egg products.
- Lacto-ovo Vegetarian: Lacto-ovo vegetarians do not consume red meat, white meat, fish, or fowl. However, lacto-ovo vegetarians do consume dairy products and egg products. This is the most common type of vegetarian.
- Nutritarians: Coined by Dr. Joel Fuhrman, this term describes his recommended lifestyle, which concentrates on eating the most micronutrient-rich foods.

According to Dr. Fuhrman, who wrote the book *Eat to Live*, and who I had the pleasure of interviewing on my show *The Raw Truth* on WDCX Radio, the quality of a diet can be based on three simple criteria:

- **Levels of micronutrients** (vitamins, minerals, phytochemicals) per calorie
- **Amounts of macronutrients** (fat, carbohydrate, protein) to meet individual needs, without excessive calories that may lead to weight gain or health compromise
- **Avoidance of potentially toxic substances** (such as trans fats) and limited amounts of other potentially harmful substances (such as sodium)

Remember that bio-individuality is key when deciding which way to go! See how your body responds to certain foods. This will require you removing some foods, then adding them back in.

I am a pescatarian, and a nutritarian, and it's been my experience in my practice that most people feel better and are healthier eating more plants than animal products. If you are a vegan or vegetarian, you need to understand that you can be vulnerable to some deficiencies like omega-3 fatty acids, iron, zinc, calcium, vitamin B-12, and vitamin D. These are all critical to your health and energy, and your mood or emotional state. If you are going to eat meat or animal products, make certain they are organic, free of hormones and antibiotics.

Protein is vital to our health, but you can eat too much protein, although I don't see this as much in my practice! Too much protein, especially animal protein, can impair our kidneys, leach calcium, zinc, vitamin B, iron, and magnesium from our bodies, and contribute to osteoporosis, heart disease, certain cancers, and obesity. Too much protein can damage our organs and accelerate aging.

Virtually everything we eat contains some protein. I'm talking greens, plant vegetables, and many fruits like bananas, blueberries, mangos, and grapes, which all contain protein.

You have probably heard that there are twenty amino acids, which are the building blocks of protein. Our bodies produce eleven, and the other nine essential amino acids can be obtained through food. There is nothing essential in meat; however, plants do contain essential vitamins, minerals, phytonutrients, and antioxidants. When you eat a well-balanced meal of whole foods, you have no problem getting your protein needs. Vitamin B-12 is important for vegetarians but they usually have no problem getting it in their diets if they are eating balanced. Yes, I know this is a mind shift for many of you but really think about it: which is better for you, plants with all the enzymes, fiber, antioxidants, and nutrients, or meat?

The choice is yours, but eat what's best for your body—and by the way, just because you are free of disease symptoms, it doesn't mean you are healthy. Most people who have a heart attack are symptom-free prior to the attack. We don't get an email, text, or phone call when we are going to have a heart attack. And no one is guaranteed tomorrow.

So, how much protein do we need? Well, that depends on how active you are and many other factors. Yes, if you are trying to build muscle, and you exercise a lot, you may need a bit more protein, but not double that of those who are sedentary.

Here's a formula that's commonly used to calculate protein needs. Divide your weight in pounds by 2.2 to get your weight in kilograms. Then plug that number into the following:

$$\text{Weight in kg} \times 0.8\text{-}1.8 \text{ gm/kg} = \text{protein gm.}$$

Use the lower number of the range if you are in good health and are sedentary (i.e., 0.8). Use the higher number (between 1 and 1.8) if you are under stress, are pregnant, are recovering from an illness, or if you are involved in consistent and intense weight or endurance training.

If you want to eat meat to get your protein, remember it's about quality not quantity, so always buy grass-fed organic. Animal protein is linked to cancer, so limit your frequency of intake. And think of your protein in terms of serving size. One serving size of meat should be no bigger than the size of the palm of your hand. Have protein and fiber with every meal to keep your blood sugar stabilized and shape your muscles lean.

Protein's Role in Building Muscle

Protein deficiency is rare, but I do see it, especially in the gym where many times it results in poor muscle tone. Often people with low-fat and/or low-protein diets have trouble losing weight and building muscle. Even if they are working out seven days a week and pumping iron many times, they still can't see muscle definition! When I finally sit down with them, nine times out of ten I find they simply lack the protein necessary in their diet to build muscle. The other problem I see is that people are either doing too much cardio, which can tear down muscle fiber, or they are using weights and resistance that are just too light for them. You need to work on the overload principle to get results! More on that in the Fitness Chapter.

CARBOHYDRATES (AND GRAINS)

Carbohydrates are important sources of vitamins, minerals, antioxidants, and fiber. If you are eating fruits and vegetables—and you should be—you also should know those are carbohydrates! I can't tell you how many times I've had people say to me, "I heard you don't eat many carbs," to which I reply, "Well, first of all, fruits and vegetables are carbs!" We know they are good for us, and I'll talk about those more in the detox section.

One of the many questions I regularly hear is, what does "other carbohydrate" mean? On the Nutrition Facts panel, "other carbohydrate" is the difference between "total carbohydrate" and the sum of dietary fiber, sugars, and sugar alcohol if declared. The difference is actually "*complex carbohydrate*," which is starch. Fiber and sugar appear as separate listings by law. Sugar includes both natural and added sugars, but you must look for added sugars on the ingredients list to tell the difference. Names for "*added sugar*" include sucrose, glucose, dextrose, honey, corn syrup, and maltodextrin to name a few. *Sugar alcohols* are listed as sorbitol, mannitol, xylitol, maltitol, and other related sugar substitutes.

Let's get into the nitty-gritty—grains!

The Good Grains: It's not about no carbs, it's about the right carbs!

We were all brought up thinking white bread is bad but wheat bread is good for us. But our wheat today is genetically modified and processed big-time, and this is wreaking havoc on our health. We now live in a processed food society, so remember it's not our grandmother's wheat anymore. It has changed, so now our mindset about wheat has to change! In fact our modern wheat (and gluten) triggers weight gain, pre-diabetes, diabetes, and more, as you will see in this section!

I truly believe that over-consumption of wheat is one of the main causes of the obesity and diabetes crisis in the United States and Canada.

Fewer than one in three Americans are of normal weight. What? That's crazy!

Remember back in the 80s when we were told to eat more healthy whole grains? How about that old food pyramid suggesting we eat six to eleven servings per day? And then there was the low-fat, eat more grain push that pushed us right into eating more processed food. And processed food is big business!

Wheat flour, cornstarch, high fructose corn syrup, sucrose, artificial sweeteners, and processed food are now the main ingredients of the products that fill the interior aisles of any modern supermarket.

We know that the increase of blood sugar and insulin are responsible for the growth of fat specifically in the visceral organs. Visceral fat, that deep fat we see around our midsection and is really around our organs as well, produces inflammation leading to diabetes, hypertension, heart disease, dementia, rheumatoid arthritis, and colon cancer at the least. That visceral fat is a special kind of fat, like an endocrine gland, much like your thyroid gland or pancreas. Visceral fat is also a factory for estrogen production in both sexes. Women then have a higher risk for breast cancer, and men develop larger breasts and also a risk of breast cancer!

High blood sugar or glucose leads to high blood insulin. High blood insulin leads to visceral fat accumulation, which causes tissues such as muscle and liver to respond less to insulin. This so-called insulin resistance means that the pancreas must produce greater and greater quantities of insulin to metabolize the sugars, eventually producing a vicious cycle of increased insulin resistance and insulin production, leading to deposits visceral fat.

As a result of this high insulin level and crazy cycle, we become increasingly hungry as the body tries to protect us from low blood sugar.

Because of wheat's ability to drive blood sugar levels up, resulting in the glucose-insulin roller coaster ride that drives appetite, generates addictive cravings, and grows visceral fat, it is one of the most important foods to eliminate for those who want to prevent or reverse diabetes or lose weight. Many of the health and fitness people I have come into contact with over my decades in the health industry think eating more grains, including wheat, is healthy! Similarly, people went on the low- or no-fat bandwagon but replaced lost fat calories with those "healthy whole grains" that have resulted in weight gain, obesity, bulging abdomens of visceral fat, pre-diabetes, and diabetes on a scale never seen before. These people are killing themselves in the gym and think they are eating healthy, but they're gaining weight! They keep doing the same things over and over, never getting results or understanding why.

Herein lies the problem. Carbohydrates trigger insulin release from the pancreas, causing growth of visceral fat; visceral fat causes insulin resistance and inflammation. High blood sugars, triglycerides, and fatty acids damage the pancreas. After years of overwork, the pancreas burns out, leaving a deficiency of insulin and an increase in blood glucose—in other words, diabetes.

What's The Big Deal about Gluten-Free?

Gluten, which comes from the Latin word for "glue," is a protein substance found in numerous grains such as wheat (which includes durum, semolina, graham, spelt, and kamut), rye, barley, and some oats since they are processed in the same machines as wheat. Used in baking, gluten gives dough its elasticity and fluffiness, and acts like glue. Gluten is everywhere. It's used in commercial soups, broths, food and spice mixes, gravy, beer, salad dressings, soy, teriyaki and other sauces, corn products, corn starch, modified starch, vegetable proteins, as an additive and stabilizing agent in many processed foods, and even in personal care products! This list isn't even complete, as it's hidden in many other products! If you have sensitivity to gluten, you need to remove it as much as possible from your diet. With celiac disease, you need to remove all of these from your diet 100%, not just the gluten-containing grains but the hidden sources as well.

The problem I see is that many people have gluten sensitivity but have never removed it from their diet to see if they are sensitive, until I do it for them. I know I was surprised early on when I found out I had sensitivity to it. Looking back now, I know it was a culprit in my failing to lose weight in my early twenties and thirties. I was brought up in a house where we had bread with every meal, and it was just the norm!

Most people recognize that gluten can be difficult to digest but don't realize that it actually can compromise our health. Gluten is commonly associated with celiac disease, but I find in my practice that more people than not have a gluten or wheat sensitivity, which wreaks havoc on their health and can sabotage their ability to lose weight, particularly around the midsection!

Gluten has the ability to permeate the gut lining, damaging the cells and allowing contents from the gut to spill into your bloodstream. Your body often attacks these (they shouldn't just be floating around in there!), causing autoimmune-like responses and inflammation in the body.

Autoimmune disorders are the number three killers, behind heart disease and cancer, in the United States. Note that gluten certainly is not always the underlying cause of all autoimmune disorders. The most common causes are food sensitivities, (not only to gluten), environmental triggers, viruses, excess estrogen exposure, and heavy metal toxicity. But it is noted that even where gluten is not the primary cause of autoimmune illness, it can almost always be suspected and eventually found as an exacerbating factor.

Gluten can affect all organs and systems in our bodies including but not limited to brain, heart, and kidneys, nervous system, digestive system, and musculoskeletal system. It affects our mood, our hormones, everything! Once food sensitivities start, if you continue to eat the foods that aggravate your body, the adverse effects are hard to reverse and can cause a vicious cycle of illnesses that gets worse with time, and is hard to reverse or manage. But you can break the chain and get help!

There is also research showing that when it comes to the effects of gluten in the brain for a gluten-sensitive person, it shuts down the blood flow to the frontal and prefrontal cortex. Gluten sensitivity has been linked to neurological disease, affecting not only the brain and nervous system, but also cognitive and mental illness. The *New England Journal of Medicine* noted that there were fifty-five diseases not just associated, but also actually caused by, gluten.

And if that's not enough for you, bread products, crackers, and pastas are making us fat! Remember, they turn into sugar and when ingested act about the same as if you had eaten a doughnut or cake. Insulin is then secreted by the pancreas, to take glucose from the blood, store it in your liver and muscles as glycogen, and stop the use of body fat for fuel. It's your fat-storage hormone.

During this period of time, your body cannot use fat for fuel (even if you are operating in a calorie deficit and even if you work out like crazy.) You can get everything else right and still sabotage yourself if you allow your insulin levels to get out of whack!

So: insulin turns off the fat-burning switch, and turns on the fat-storage switch. And then you crave more junk! Does this sound like you? It was me as well, back in the day!

Deep visceral fat accumulation, particularly in the midsection, results from years of consuming foods that trigger insulin, the hormone of fat storage. Unlike fat in other body areas, it stimulates an inflammatory process, distorts insulin responses, and issues abnormal metabolic signals to the rest of the body. This is a problem!

On top of that, people overeat because their food isn't real food and their hormones, like leptin, increase their appetite. But taste buds can change with a detox! For most Americans and Canadians, every single meal and snack contains foods made with wheat flour.

Wheat, by a considerable margin, is the dominant source of gluten protein in the human diet.

In my practice, after removing gluten and grains for just thirty to ninety days from the diets of my diabetic/overweight patients, the diabetics became *non*-diabetic and many of them had lost twenty, thirty, forty, even fifty pounds!

Additionally for these people, acid reflux disappeared, cramping and diarrhea stopped, energy and focus improved, sleep was deeper, rashes disappeared, rheumatoid arthritis pain improved, and asthma symptoms improved.

- Glucose is accompanied by insulin, the hormone that allows entry of glucose into the cells of the body, converting the glucose to fat. Aside from the benefits of some fiber, eating two slices of whole-wheat bread acts about the same as drinking a can of sugar-sweetened soda or eating a sugary candy bar.

- The higher the blood glucose after consumption of food, the greater the insulin level, and the more fat is deposited, particularly in the midsection as deep visceral fat. Do you see why eating protein would be a much better choice when you're hungry?

- It's no surprise that when people omit wheat products from their diet they experience withdrawal symptoms: fatigue, mental fog, irritability, inability to function at work or school, depression. The result is that we want more bad carbs and wheat-containing foods, and it's a vicious cycle again!

- If you have never done a detox like The Raw Truth Recharge you probably find it hard to imagine that wheat, sugar, and caffeine can affect the central nervous system as much as nicotine or crack cocaine do.

Celiac Disease

The most dramatic evidence of failed adaptation to wheat is celiac disease, the disruption of small intestinal health by wheat gluten. So many patients with celiac disease are misdiagnosed with diarrhea.

There are plenty of gluten-free substitutes out there, and it's a big business, as you know! Even gluten-free cosmetics and shampoos are available. But you should know that even though other grains, such as quinoa, buckwheat, soy, millet, and rice don't technically contain gluten, these foods many times are contaminated, and to me ingesting gluten or grains of any kind is somewhat of a risk that may not be worth it in the end.

But don't we need grains? There is no research that shows that grains of any kind are essential for health, and gluten in particular definitely is not. I like to stick to foods of the earth we don't need to read a label on! The Raw Truth is that it's less confusing, less complicated and better for us in the long run.

Bottom line, my friends: you will drop weight drastically when you eliminate wheat and other gluten-containing grains, like barley and rye, from your diet. You need to control and manage the amount of carbohydrate and sugars in your diet to your own individual tolerance levels, which in turn will stabilize your blood sugars and help you lose weight. This is where bio-individuality once again comes in.

I don't know about you, but all this is enough for me to want to stay away from gluten forever! The good news is that the devastating symptoms and illness associated with gluten sensitivity and celiac disease can be avoided and eliminated entirely!

Quinoa

A lot of vegetarians and people who want to lose weight have turned to quinoa (pronounced KEEN-wah) because it's high in protein and fiber, and low in the glycemic index. It is a relative of beets, chard, and spinach. The seed can be prepared just like many whole grains, and most recipes for quinoa treat it much like any other grain. Quinoa is mild and slightly nutty, similar to couscous but not exactly the same.

Quinoa is a great food for people who must follow wheat-free/gluten-free diets because quinoa doesn't contain gluten. And it's a nutritional powerhouse! Quinoa is loaded with vitamins and minerals. The fact that it contains magnesium, copper, and phosphorus means that quinoa is especially good for those who have migraine headaches, atherosclerosis, and diabetes. Quinoa is a great source of healthy carbohydrates, and it also provides five grams of fiber and eight grams of protein per serving. It couldn't be more perfect for those of us who want a lot of energy but don't want to pack on the pounds!

According to The National Academy of Sciences, quinoa is "one of the best sources of protein in the vegetable kingdom." Quinoa contains the amino acid lysine, which helps the body produce protein. It also helps the body process the protein in the quinoa and in other foods. The World Health Organization has rated the quality of protein in quinoa to be equivalent or superior to that found in milk products.

Quinoa is a source of all essential amino acids, according to the United Nations Food and Agricultural Organization.

It's a great source of B vitamins, containing niacin, thiamin, and B-6. It contains high levels of potassium and riboflavin. It's also a good source of zinc, copper, manganese, and magnesium. It contains folic acid and vitamin E.

Sprouted Grains

The Food for Life Baking Company's Ezekiel 4:9 products are my favorite sprouted-grain products, and not just because the recipe is in the Bible (but that's a good reason)!

> *Take also unto thee wheat, and barley, and beans, and lentils and millet, and spelt and put them in one vessel… Ezekiel 4:9*

Their breads, pastas, cereals, and other foods contain a unique combination of six grains and legumes, and they are a great source of complete protein. They also contain eighteen amino acids, including all nine essential amino acids, and they are easy to digest, as sprouting breaks down starches in grains into simple sugars so your body can digest them easily. Sprouting also helps with the absorption of minerals, because it breaks down enzyme inhibitors, so your body can more easily absorb calcium, magnesium, iron, copper, and zinc. It also produces vitamin C and increases vitamins B-2, B-5 and B-6. Finally, the sprouted products are a great source of fiber.

Not all whole grains are healthy. But if you find non-GMO organic whole grains, they could be good for you. Whole grains contain all parts of the grain, including the bran, endosperm, and germ. If you choose to go gluten-free, make sure your products are organic, non-GMO, and not processed with preservatives.

Whole Grain Truths

- Choose organic whole grains with at least five grams of fiber per serving.
- Choose organic cereals made primarily of oats, barley, and bran for breakfast or a snack. Be aware that most cereals are high-glycemic.
- Use whole-grain bread. I prefer Ezekiel 4:9 Sprouted Grain breads, which are high in protein and fiber and flourless.
- Eat black or brown rice instead of white rice, and use quinoa.
- Experiment with cooking various whole grains like barley and millet.
- When buying bread products, read the label. Look for items labeled "100% Organic Whole Grain" to ensure you are truly buying a whole-grain product.

- Know that wheat flour and whole-wheat flour are not the same! Look for whole grain, stone ground, whole ground, whole-wheat flour, whole-oat flour or whole-barley flour.
- When eating a refined grain, add foods with plenty of fiber (fruits, vegetables, and legumes) to lower the glycemic impact.
- Be aware of high-glycemic breads and bagels. Try hemp breads, which are high in protein and fiber.
- Use steel-cut oats rather than other oats. They are lower in the glycemic index compared to regular oats. They are high in fiber and protein and low in fat. They are very nutritiously dense.
- Choose gluten-free if you have a gluten sensitivity or celiac disease. But know that just because something is gluten-free doesn't mean it's low-glycemic or that it contains other good ingredients.
- Stay away from processed or refined grains including bleached and enriched.

FATS

There are many types of fat. Your body makes its own fat from taking in excess calories, and that can come from having too much of anything. Some fats are found in foods from plants and animals and are known as dietary fat. Dietary fat is a macronutrient that provides energy for your body. Fat is essential to your health because it supports a number of your body's functions. Some vitamins, for instance, must have fat to dissolve and nourish your body. Your brain needs fat.

But there is a dark side to fat. Fat is high in calories, and small amounts can add up quickly. Having nuts is better than having oils, though. Nuts and seeds take three to four hours to digest. Too much oil could be a problem in weight loss, so don't overdo it!

Fat is Not the Enemy

For years we thought if you wanted to lose weight you needed to eat fat-free foods. Do you remember the fat-free era? We were cutting fat grams to lose weight, and it was fat-free this and fat-free that. The result was that everyone got fatter, and obesity rates escalated, as well as cholesterol levels! Why? Because we took the fat out of the food and put sugar and processed ingredients in!

Most of the clients I have seen who avoid fat to lose weight are some of the most unhealthy people on the planet. And the truth is, adding good fats to your diet does not make you fat! And low-fat diets actually make us hungry! I myself used to think I could eat as many fat-free cookies as I wanted back in my unhealthy days because they were fat-free! If you don't get enough fat in your diet, you will never feel completely satisfied, and you will end up overeating.

Combine that with the fact that the low-fat, high-sugar stuff makes us crave more junk! Low fat usually means high carbohydrate. And high carbs lead to low blood sugar. When your blood sugar drops, your body goes into storage mode and your metabolism slows down. That's just the way God made us, with a built-in self-defense mechanism. And when your blood sugar drops, so does your energy to function with daily activities, and then exercise is a distant memory.

Including good fats with every meal helps keep your blood sugar stabilized and your metabolism up, by providing your body with a steady supply of fuel (food) to burn throughout the day.

In fact, you don't even need to feel guilty about eating good fat, because it is essential to our health! The human brain is made up of 65% fats, our hormones are made from fat, and so is the outer layer of the cells in our body. Fats stabilize our blood sugar, keep our skin looking healthy and youthful, prevent diabetes, enhance our immune system, normalize our cholesterol, benefit our hearts (and brains), and even help prevent cancer!

A deficiency of fat can lead to fatigue, depression, anxiety, mood swings, hypoglycemia, extreme hunger and cravings, hormonal imbalances, gall bladder problems, inability to concentrate, memory loss, bloating, and even lack of menstruation in young women. Lack of healthy fat in the diet can cause your nails and hair to be dry and brittle, and your skin to look aged.

The Good Fats:

Monounsaturated fat. Olive oil, avocado, and most nuts. Eat these! (In fact, studies have linked them to fat loss.)

Polyunsaturated fat, such as omega-3 from fish oils, salmon, trout, and omega-6 fats from vegetable oils. Our bodies can't make these essential fatty acids—we must get them from food.

Good for you oils are extra-virgin olive oil, coconut oil, hemp oil, walnut, almond oil, peanut oil, macadamia oil, red palm oil, and sesame oil. (Cold-pressed is always best).

Trans fats are the real villain, causing far more significant health problems than saturated fat.

Harmful dietary fat

There are two main types of potentially harmful dietary fat—fat that is mostly saturated and fat that contains trans fat:

- **Saturated fat.** This type of fat comes mainly from animal sources of food, such as red meat, poultry, and full-fat dairy products. Saturated fat raises total blood cholesterol levels and low-density lipoprotein (LDL) cholesterol levels, which can increase your risk of cardiovascular disease. Saturated fat may also increase your risk of type 2 diabetes.
- **Trans fat.** This type of fat occurs naturally in some foods in small amounts. But most trans fats are made from oils through a food processing method called partial hydrogenation. Partially hydrogenating oils makes them easier to cook with and less likely to spoil than do naturally occurring oils. Research studies show that these partially hydrogenated trans fats can increase unhealthy LDL cholesterol and lower healthy high-density lipoprotein (HDL) cholesterol.

Stay away from cottonseed oil, canola oil, vegetable oil, rapeseed oil, soybean oil, corn oil, hydrogenated, and partially hydrogenated oil.

Here are 7 Raw Truths about Fats:

1) Choose organic butter, not margarine. Butter is a rich source of fat-soluble vitamins, including A, D, E, and K.
2) Use traditional fats, not processed vegetable oils.

3) Avoid reduced- and zero-fat products. These are food-like things, not food.

4) Use organic cold pressed extra virgin olive oil (EVOO). Olive oil is rich in antioxidants, normalizes blood fats and cholesterol, relieves the pain and inflammation of arthritis, and is known to increase longevity.

5) Use organic coconut (and palm oils). I could do a whole chapter on coconut oil, but here's the 411!

- Studies have shown that an intake of coconut oil can help our bodies increase resistance to both viruses and bacteria that can cause illness. Even more, it can help to fight off yeast, fungus, and candida. It can also have a positive effect on our cholesterol.

- It can positively affect our hormones for thyroid and blood sugar control by helping improve insulin use in the body. It can boost thyroid function, helping to increase metabolism, energy, and endurance. It increases digestion and helps to absorb fat-soluble vitamins.

- Coconut oil can help keep weight balanced, and research shows that it can actually help reduce abdominal fat.

6) Organic raw nuts are great for you although you should watch your portion sizes!

- Raw macadamia nuts are a powerhouse of a nut, containing a wide variety of critical nutrients including high amounts of vitamin B-1, magnesium, manganese, and healthful monounsaturated fat, just to name a few.

- Raw walnuts are good sources of plant-based omega-3 fats and antioxidants. Walnuts may help reduce not only the risk of prostate cancer, but breast cancer as well. They've also been shown to reverse brain aging in rats and boost heart health in people with diabetes.

- Raw almonds: One of the healthiest aspects of almonds appears to be their skins, as they are rich in antioxidants, which are typically associated with vegetables and fruits. A study in the *Journal of Agricultural and Food Chemistry* even revealed that a one-ounce serving of almonds has similar benefits as a cup of steamed broccoli or green tea.

- Pecans contain more than nineteen vitamins and minerals, and research has shown they may help lower LDL cholesterol and promote healthy arteries.
- Brazil nuts: Brazil nuts are an excellent source of organic selenium, a powerful antioxidant-boosting mineral that may help prevent cancer.

7) Avocados are high in fat, but they are monounsaturated fat, which is a "good" fat that helps lower bad cholesterol, as long as you eat it in moderation. Avocados offer nearly twenty vitamins and minerals in every serving, including potassium (which helps control blood pressure), lutein (which is good for your eyes), and folate (which is crucial for cell repair and during pregnancy). Avocados are a good source of B vitamins, which help you fight off disease and infection. They also give you vitamins C and E, plus natural plant chemicals that may help prevent cancer.

Milk Madness

I was brought up drinking milk, just like many of you. Over the years I switched to soy milk, which both my kids were brought up on, and then I made the switch years ago to unsweetened almond milk, which we all drink now. My dear Mom (God bless her), and many other people I come across still can't understand how we can survive without cow's milk. Here are the facts—you decide, by comparing a one-cup serving of the following:

Beverage	Calories	Fat grams	Sugar grams	Vitamin D	Calcium
Cow's milk	130	5	12	25%	30%
Coconut milk	80	5	6	30%	10%
Rice milk	120	2.5	10	25%	30%
Soy milk	90	3.5	6	30%	30%
Unsweetened almond milk	60	2.5	<1	25%	30%

Almond milk is also a great source of antioxidants and vitamins A and E, it's gluten and lactose-free, and it tastes delicious!!

Great sources of Calcium, or What the National Dairy Council Does Not Want You To Know

- Fortified cereals
- Fortified orange juice
- Tofu, soy milk and tempeh
- Collards
- Kale
- Edamame
- Sesame seeds
- Fortified almond milk
- Rice milk

Your Daily Intake of Macronutrients

Protein:
10-35% of your daily intake should be from protein, about forty-five to sixty-five grams of protein per day for general health. Remember, you need protein to maintain tissue and muscle. If you don't get enough protein, your muscles will break down to supply it. You don't need animal products to get in protein, although it is certainly easier if you are body building and your protein needs are higher.

Fats:
The type of fat you consume makes all the difference to your health. The daily recommended intake of fat is twenty to thirty percent of your total daily calorie intake, with saturated fats and trans fats kept to less than ten percent of your total intake.

Carbohydrates:
Men and women of all ages should get about 45 to 65 % of their total daily calories from carbohydrates.

Ingredients

The ingredients you see listed on any type of processed food are listed in order of quantity, but that doesn't always tell the whole story. For example, if a jar of salsa lists tomatoes first, you know there are more tomatoes in the product than anything else. But when it comes to sodium, added sugars, and saturated and trans fats—which in excess can damage your heart health and increase your risk of heart disease and stroke—it can be difficult to tell just how much is in there. The reason is, these ingredients can go by several names.

You might see sugar listed as the fourth ingredient in a product and think it's not so bad. But sugar can also be listed as high-fructose corn syrup or corn syrup, agave nectar, barley malt syrup or dehydrated cane juice, to name just a few. Other names for added sugar include sucrose, glucose, dextrose, honey, and maltodextrin. Sugar alcohols are listed as sorbitol, mannitol, xylitol, maltitol, and other related sugar substitutes.

On the Nutrition Facts panel, "other carbohydrate" is the difference between "total carbohydrate" and the sum of dietary fiber, sugars, and sugar alcohol if declared. Sugar includes both natural and added sugars but you must look for added sugars on the ingredients list to tell the difference. Microminerals or trace elements include at least iron, cobalt, chromium, copper, iodine, manganese, selenium, zinc and molybdenum. **Micronutrients** also include vitamins, which are organic compounds required as nutrients in tiny amounts by an organism. Micronutrients are different from macronutrients (like carbohydrates, protein and fat) because they are necessary only in very tiny amounts. Nevertheless, micronutrients are essential for good health, and micronutrient deficiencies can cause serious health problems. We won't get into all of that here, but you should take vitamins, which I will mention later.

GMOs or GEs

Seventy percent of our processed foods contain either corn or soy and contain at least one genetically modified ingredient. A genetically modified organism (GMO) or genetically engineered (GE) is a plant or an animal that has had DNA genes from another organism artificially forced into its own DNA. These products are engineered in a laboratory using highly complex technology, such as gene splicing. The foreign genes come from bacteria, viruses, insects, and animals. The goal of mixing the genes together is to create stronger crops and increase pest resistance.

We know a lot about the toxins sprayed on GMO crops and how they adversely affect our health. For years, Monsanto has sold its flagship weed killer product, called Roundup, to farmers and consumers worldwide. This stuff kills weeds while allowing GMO crops to thrive, and more chemicals to infiltrate our foods. Did you know that any time you eat corn you are probably consuming a dose of Roundup with it? And the result, as noted in the journal *Food and Chemical Toxicology* in 2012, is serious long-term health problems ranging from breast cancer to endocrine disorders and everything in between.

We need laws requiring labeling of foods with GMO ingredients. Currently sixty-four countries regulate their GMO foods, but the United States does not.

GMO crops currently being developed are corn, soy, canola, cotton, sugar beets, yellow squash, zucchini, Hawaiian papaya, and alfalfa. So avoid anything that shows the following in the label: soybean oil, canola oil, cottonseed oil, or corn syrup and corn products. Also stay clear of nonorganic flax, rice, and wheat, as these also may have been contaminated with pesticides.

Any food labeled as USDA Organic should not have any GMOs in any of its ingredients. The key phrase is "should not," so make sure you are getting it from a reputable source. Equally important to note is that just because something is labeled non-GMO does not mean it is organic!

The Non-GMO Project (www.nongmoproject.org) is the only organization offering independent verification of testing and GMO controls for products in the United States and Canada.

Bottom line, avoid all non-organic produce and foods, and always read the label. And by the way, if you stop eating processed foods, you won't need to worry about GMOs much.

How to Read a Produce Label

The produce lookup (PLU) code is the number the cashier punches into the register to identify the fruits or vegetables you buy. And the PLU code can tell you if the produce is organically grown, conventionally grown or genetically modified and could cause sickness and disease.

- If there are only four digits in the PLU, this means that the produce was grown conventionally or "traditionally," with the use of pesticides. For example, traditionally grown bananas will be labeled with the code of 4011.
- If there are five digits in the PLU, starting with the numeral 8, this means it is a GMO and should be avoided at all costs! A genetically engineered (GE or GMO) banana would be labeled with the code 84011.
- If there are five digits in the PLU starting with the numeral 9, this means it is organically grown and not genetically modified. And that's what you want! The produce has been grown using no synthetic fertilizers or pesticides. An organic banana would be labeled with the code 94011.

The Dirty Dozen Plus
The USDA found more than fifty pesticide residues on fruits and veggies that range from carcinogens to chemicals that cause blurred vision, rashes, asthma, thyroid issues and reproductive and developmental damage. The produce that is rated highest in contamination for pesticides are called the Dirty Dozen:

1. apples
2. strawberries
3. grapes
4. celery
5. peaches
6. spinach
7. sweet bell peppers
8. nectarines (imported)
9. cucumbers
10. cherry tomatoes
11. snap peas (imported)
12. potatoes
+ hot peppers
+ kale/collard greens

(Kale, collard greens, and hot peppers were frequently contaminated with insecticides that are particularly toxic to human health, prompting their "Dirty Dozen Plus" status.)

The Clean 15

It's not all bad news! These produce picks contained the lowest pesticide levels:

- avocados
- sweet corn (but watch for GMO)
- pineapples
- cabbage
- sweet peas (frozen)
- onions
- asparagus
- mangoes
- papayas
- eggplant
- kiwi
- grapefruit
- cantaloupe
- cauliflower
- sweet potatoes

Fruit and Vegetable Washes

You can purchase fruit and vegetable washes at your local store. Make sure you scrub your produce with a vegetable brush and soak if at all possible. Or, you can make your own:

Homemade Vegetable/Fruit
Wash 1 Tbsp. lemon juice
2 Tbsp. baking soda
1 Tbsp. grape seed extract
¾ cup of vinegar
8 oz. of water

Pour the solution into a spray bottle and spray your produce. Let the solution sit on your fruits and veggies for about 5 minutes before rinsing it off under cool water.

Phytonutrients

It's important to note that more than 25,000 phytonutrients (also known as phytochemicals) are found in plant foods (fruits, vegetables, nuts, beans, tea, whole grains). Phytonutrients aren't essential for keeping you alive, unlike the vitamins and minerals that plant foods contain. But when you eat or drink phytonutrients, they may help prevent disease and keep your body working properly.

Sodium: How much do you need?

There's salt, sodium benzoate, disodium or monosodium glutamate (MSG). It's in lunch meats, used to preserve fish and meats, and control bacteria, so it has legitimate uses, but we should be aware of how sodium contributes to our total salt intake.

This is important to know because too much sodium can raise blood pressure, increasing risk for heart disease and stroke. The American Heart Association recommends no more than 1,500 milligrams of sodium a day, but the average American consumes twice that much. With that said, many experts now believe the former guidelines are antiquated and if your body is craving salt you should have it. In fact studies show that a lack of salt in the diet can <u>cause</u> a cardiac event.

Bottom line is, salt is essential for life, meaning you cannot live without it. However, most people simply don't realize that there are enormous differences between the standard, refined table and cooking salt most of you are accustomed to using, and natural, healthy salt. I prefer unrefined Redmond Real Salt or Pink Himalayan Salt.

- Don't exceed 2,300 mg of sodium a day if you're a healthy adult.
- Don't exceed 1,500 mg of sodium a day if you have high blood pressure, kidney disease or diabetes; or if you're middle-aged or older.

Keep in mind that athletes need much more. If you aren't sure how much sodium your diet should include, talk to your doctor or health practitioner.

Main dietary sources

To help keep your sodium consumption in check, you need to know where the sodium comes from. Here are the main sources of sodium in a typical diet:

- **Processed and prepared foods.** You need to avoid processed food for many reasons, and here is yet another one. The vast majority of dietary sodium comes from eating foods that are processed and prepared. These foods are typically high in salt, which is a combination of sodium and chloride, and in additives that contain sodium. While these ingredients have many practical uses—such as preservation and enhanced taste—they can greatly increase your sodium intake.
- **Natural sources.** Some foods naturally contain sodium. These include celery and some other vegetables, dairy products such as milk, and meat and shellfish. While they don't have an abundance of sodium, eating these foods does add to your overall sodium intake.
- **In the kitchen and at the table.** Many recipes call for salt, and many people also salt their food at the table. And many other condiments also contain sodium. If you are going to add it, stick with Redmond Real Salt or Himalayan salt, which are much better for you.

The Sweet Stuff

You don't have to give up all sweets. It's all about the ingredients! The "bad" sugars (below) and foods with added sugars not only will cause depression, irritability, mood swings, premature aging, and low energy, but they will make us fat, particularly around the midsection! Sugar is just empty calories with no nutritional value, which messes up with your appetite controls and causes your blood sugar to skyrocket, then crash and burn. Too much sugar has been linked to cognitive declines; it can negatively affect our immune system, and ruin our health. And did you know that cancer has a sweet tooth? It also makes your body more acidic. Stay away from the stuff and anything that has added sugar. It's an addictive toxin that you will need to detox from if you ever want to break the chain.

As for the "bad" sugars:

- Avoid all sugars, hidden sugars and any products that contain the following ingredients: fructose, brown sugar, high fructose corn syrup, turbinado sugar, sucrose, agave, barley malt, carob, caramel, agave nectar, beet sugar, invert sugar, dextrose, dextran, diastase, glucose, and raw sugar.
- Avoid all artificial sweeteners and any products that contain the following ingredients: aspartame, saccharin, or sucralose (Splenda). These cause a variety of health problems and some have been linked to cancer. In my thirty-year career, I have never seen anyone get thin using artificial ingredients. In fact, most overweight people are drinking diet pop, which contains aspartame. Not only is aspartame linked to health problems, but it causes you to crave more sweet stuff.

I still like to have my treats once in a while, but I don't crave them anymore, and the kind I have doesn't make me go off the train rail so much I go into a train wreck! So, the key is to have the good sweeteners. Remember, you crave what you eat, and you eat what you crave.

The "Good" Sweeteners
You can eat these, but limit yourself!

- Coconut nectar and coconut palm sugar come from the coconut palm tree flowers. It's a natural unprocessed sugar, which is lower in the glycemic index, is great for baking and measures the same as sugar. (Anything that comes from a palm tree is all right with me)!
- Stevia comes from the stevia plant and doesn't contain any calories. Look for "whole leaf" stevia. Do not be fooled by imitations that are processed and contain other unfavorable ingredients.
- Honey is the least refined sweetener in the world. It isn't low glycemic, but it does have several health benefits. It contains antioxidants and is known to activate serotonin, which can lift your mood and promote better sleep.
- Real maple syrup, the kind that comes right from the maple tree, is loaded with antioxidants, vitamins, minerals, and amino acids. It is not low glycemic, however.

The Body's pH

There is a method to my madness, and it's not just about your waistline! Eating more alkaline foods will maximize your health. A more acidic environment opens the door and accelerates the rate of cancer spreading in the body and illness; a more alkaline environment inhibits the chance and the spread of cancer. In fact, cancer cannot survive in an oxygenated alkaline environment. Too much sugar, dairy, animal products, and junk food increases your body's acidity. Fruits and vegetables contribute to a more alkaline state.

pH Balance
The pH scale goes from 0-14
The numbers below 7 are acidic (low oxygen)
The numbers above 7 are alkaline.

Blood, lymph, and cerebral spinal fluid in the body are designed to be slightly alkaline at a pH of 7.4.

If your body's pH goes too high or too low, from the normal pH of 7.4 by just .5, you could die!

- Acids drive pH down, triggering a response from the body to try and compensate. The body responds by drawing from any alkaline store available, from the bloodstream and the bones.
- The body is happier and healthier being slightly more alkaline.
- Major dietary source of acid: carbonated sodas, junk food, and any foods derived from animal sources generate some acid challenge.

Vegetables and fruits are the dominant alkaline foods in the diet. At least 60-80% of your diet should be alkaline. Acidic diets eat up your minerals, alkalizing diets replenish your minerals. Minerals help your body to build essentials to its health; proteins enzymes, hormones, etc. Foods that are high in minerals are high in alkaline.

A diet of "healthy whole grains" but lacking in vegetables and fruit is highly acid-charged, inducing a condition called acidosis, which takes a toll on your bones. Grains are the only plant product that generate acidic by-products.

Avoid:
Beef, cheese, whey protein, isolated soy protein, pork, milk, coffee, sugar, margarine, roasted nuts, synthetic supplements to name a few.

In Summary
Illness and disease can be caused by acidification. Balancing your alkaline and acidic levels is a big key to health. Know that exercise improves your pH balance!

Water
You probably have heard that our bodies are 70% water, but did you know that our brain is more than 80% water and our blood is more than 90% water? Right there is a good reason why you should drink water, so go get some right now!

Most people don't drink enough water. Many people are also carrying around a few more pounds than they would be if they did drink enough water. If you can't seem to get that weight off, it may be because you are dehydrated. Being dehydrated slows down your metabolic rate, which decreases your energy level and ability to burn fat. Just what you want, right? Wrong!

If you're trying to lose weight and burn fat, make sure that you are hydrated. Your body needs a healthy functioning metabolism to do that, and if your metabolism is slow because you are dehydrated, that doesn't help things much. Water also improves muscle tone, plumps up your muscles, and helps your skin look more youthful!

One of the liver's duties is to help out the kidneys when needed. Your kidneys need plenty of water to work properly. If the kidneys are water-deprived, the liver has to do their work along with its own, lowering its total productivity. The liver then can't metabolize fat as quickly or efficiently as it could when the kidneys were pulling their own weight. This will cause your body to store fat. Not good.

Fluctuating blood sugar levels or elevated blood sugar in association with excess body weight are predictive of a clogged liver. Conversely, when you are able to eat a normal amount of carbohydrates and not gain weight from them, your liver is functioning better. When your liver is clogged with fat, it has difficulty breaking down fat to use as fuel. Your liver and white adipose tissue are constantly breaking down and restoring fat (triglycerides).

The problem is that once the liver is clogged, then the process becomes imbalanced and tilts more toward fat storage than fat breakdown. This shows up in elevated triglycerides in your blood and weight gain. Have I convinced you yet?

How Much Water Should You Drink?

Divide your weight in pounds by 2 and drink that many ounces of water per day just to sustain life. If you weigh 150 pounds, divide by two and drink 75 ounces per day minimum (10 cups). Eight 8-ounce glasses of water, or about two quarts, is the general recommendation and okay for the average person. But this general recommendation is not taking into account bio-individuality, like if you're overweight, exercising, living in a hot climate, are sick, or go in the sauna, which are times when you should drink more. Of course not everyone weighs the same so their water consumption shouldn't be the same. Your water consumption should be spread out throughout the day. It's not healthy at all to drink too much water at one time. Don't let yourself get thirsty, however. If you feel thirsty, you've already become dehydrated. Drink when you're not thirsty yet.

When you start drinking a lot of water, you feel as if it's going right through you. What is really happening is that your body is flushing itself of the water it has been storing throughout all those years of "survival mode." It takes a while, but this is a beautiful thing happening to you. As you continue to give your body all the water it could ask for, it gets rid of what it doesn't need. It gets rid of the water it was holding onto in your ankles and your hips and thighs, maybe even around your belly. You are excreting much more than you realize. Your body figures it doesn't need to save the stored-up water anymore; it's trusting that the water will keep coming, and if it does, eventually, the flushing out (also known as detoxing) will cease. This is called the "breakthrough point."

Caffeine should not take the place of water. You should be aware of the fact that many people like caffeine because it's known to increase the body's fat-burning potential slightly. This finding may hold some degree of truth in it, but caffeine is also a diuretic, and diuretics dehydrate. Caffeine may increase the heart rate, causing a few more calories to be burned, but this is at the expense of the muscles, which need water to function properly.

Caffeine also affects your blood sugar, which could cause you to crave sweets.

Bottom line, if you are trying to be healthy, feel great, or lose weight, it's paramount that you drink enough water. If you don't like the taste of water (although it shouldn't have any taste) than put some lemon, lime, cucumbers, strawberries, or ginger in it, but drink!

Filter Your Water!

You can eat all the best organic foods on the entire planet but be drinking water with toxins in it and be incredibly sick and unhealthy!

What's happening in our food supply is bad, but equally bad is what's happening with our water supply! I don't have to tell you that drinking clean, uncontaminated water is vital to your health. There are toxins in the air, the food, the water and the soil.

In 2010, the Environmental Working Group, a nonpartisan, nonprofit organization reported that tap water they tested from forty-five states contained over 300 contaminants! Those contaminants included but were not limited to radon, a radioactive gas; Freon, a refrigerant pumped into air conditioners; the weed killer metolachlor; and acetone, the liquid used to remove nail polish.

Some other contaminants in our tap water include aluminum, arsenic, chlorine, chromium, fluoride, gas, oil, lead, microbes, nitrates, perchlorate, pesticides, and prescription drugs. You don't need to be a rocket scientist to know these aren't good for your health!

You need to filter your drinking water and your shower water, too, as our skin is the largest organ in the body.

The Raw Truth is this:

1) Get a good water and shower filter that filters out the above contaminants.
2) Drink water out of a glass or stainless steel bottle.
3) If you are using plastic bottles, it's important to be aware of the risks they pose.

This can be determined through a classification system called the Resin Identification Code, which is the number printed on the bottom of most plastic bottles and food containers. It describes what kind of plastic resin the product is made out of. So check the number on the bottom. Those that contain the #2, #4 and #5 are generally considered *somewhat safer*. Plastic #1 is safer too but should not be re-used due to the risk of growing bacteria.

Any other plastic should be used with extreme caution, especially around food or drink, if they have a #3, #6 or #7. The risk is even greater when heating food. For microwaving in particular, remember that microwave-safe containers aren't necessarily healthy. They just won't melt. In general, it's better to avoid microwaving plastic entirely and stick to glass. In fact, to be really safe, throw the microwave out with the plastic bottles!

My Favorite Superfoods and Drinks!

The food from the earth is a gift from God, and sometimes we take for granted the incredible benefits of some of the most basic common foods from our earth. Although this list is constantly changing, here are some of my favorites foods and drinks that heal and fuel our bodies:

- **Beets:** Contain folate, fiber, and potassium. The greens are a great source of Vitamin C, calcium, iron and beta-carotene. Helps lower the risk of heart disease.
- **Onions and Garlic:** Stimulate the immunes system's natural defenses against cancer and may have the potential to decrease tumor growth. May help prevent blood clots and lower blood pressure.
- **Green Tea:** A great antioxidant. Helps with fat burning. May help reduce the formation of carcinogens in the body and increase the body's natural defenses. An immune booster that contains antioxidants called catechins, which may inhibit the growth of cancer cells and also may help reduce cholesterol. My favorite is matcha green tea. Used for increased focus, energy, and metabolism to name a few.
- **Broccoli:** Great source of fiber, vitamin C, beta carotene, protein, calcium, potassium, iron and other minerals. Cancer-fighting, as is cauliflower.
- **Good fats:** Olive oil, coconut oil, walnut oil, nuts (especially almonds and walnuts), and seeds, fatty fish (deep wild salmon), avocados, flaxseed oil, chia seeds. Good for growth and development

and brain function; protect the heart; lower triglycerides; help prevent blood clotting.

- **Cold-Pressed Extra-Virgin Olive Oil**: Protects against heart disease by reducing LDL (bad) cholesterol and raising good HDL cholesterol.
- **Beans/Legumes**: Contain more protein than any other plant. Contains Vitamin B complex, iron, potassium, zinc, and other essential minerals. High fiber.
- **Leafy Green Veggies** (Romaine, Arugula, Endive, Kale, Escarole): Contain beta-carotene, folate, vitamin C, calcium, iron and potassium.
- **Spinach**: Great source of folate, Vitamins A (as beta carotene), and C, riboflavin, potassium. Folate deficiency can cause a severe type of anemia. Folate is also important for pregnant women to help prevent birth defects.
- **Strawberries**: Excellent source of Vitamin C. Good source of pectin and other soluble fibers that help lower cholesterol. Contains folate and potassium. Anti-cancer.
- **Blueberries**: Help prevent urinary tract infections (UTIs). Great antioxidant, fiber, Vitamin C, iron, may help with memory loss, and heart disease. Cranberries also help prevent UTIs and cancer.
- **Grapefruit**: Lowers levels of cancer-causing enzymes and a great source of vitamin C.
- **Wild Salmon**: A healthy fat, which raises good HDL cholesterol levels. Also contains omega-3 fatty acids, which help fight heart disease.
- **Raspberries**: Contain anthocyanins, which boost insulin production and lower blood sugar levels. All deep-colored berries (blue, red, purple, black) contain the highest levels of antioxidants and vitamins of any fruits. They strengthen the immune system, help prevent cancer and prevent cell damage, and may improve brain function.
- **Pomegranate**: Reduces bad LDL cholesterol and heart disease risk and may help prevent osteoporosis.
- **Broccoli**: Rich in vitamin C and cancer-fighting.

- **Raw Shelled Hemp Seeds**: They contain 10 grams of omegas 3 and 6 and are an excellent source of protein, with ten grams in three tablespoons.
- **Chia Seeds and Flax Seeds**: As an athlete, I prefer chia seeds over flax seeds because they retain water and help keep me hydrated. They also don't need to be ground up.
- **Raw Maca Powder**: Used for energy, balance, and vitality. Contains four alkaloids known to nourish the endocrine system. Used to increase stamina, boost libido, and combat fatigue. Maca is a nutrient-dense food packed with vitamins, plant sterols as well as many essential minerals, fatty and amino acids. *Maca is contraindicated for people who are pregnant, nursing, have thyroid conditions, or other conditions.*
- **Bragg's Organic Raw Apple Cider Vinegar**: Rich in enzymes and potassium. Supports a healthy immune system. Helps control weight. Promotes digestion and pH balance. Helps remove toxins. Helps promote youthful healthy bodies.
- **Bragg's Liquid Aminos**: Bragg's Liquid Aminos is a certified, non-GMO liquid protein concentrate, derived from healthy soybeans, that contains essential and non-essential amino acids in naturally occurring amounts.
- **Coconut Oil:** A heart-healthy food that has so many benefits we can't list them all. Used for everything from hair and skin products to a healthy body and immune system! Even more, it is used to fight off yeast, fungus, and candida. Coconut oil can also positively affect our hormones for thyroid and blood sugar control. Used to stabilize blood sugar and improve insulin use within the body. Coconut oil is used to boost thyroid function, helping to increase metabolism, energy, and endurance. It increases digestion and helps to absorb fat-soluble vitamins. Obviously a whole coconut and flakes are a great way to snack!
- **Aloe Juice:** Over 200 nutrients and used to boost the immune system and many other health benefits. Helps heal mucus membranes.
- **Raw Cacao Powder and Nibs:** Help increase energy and enhance health. These babies are high in fiber, iron and magnesium, and many other essential minerals.

- **Kombucha:** Loaded with enzymes and used to boost immune system and many other health benefits.
- **Shiitake Mushrooms:** Used to fight the development and progression of cancer and AIDS by boosting the body's immune system. These mushrooms are also said to help prevent heart disease by lowering cholesterol levels. Also used to help treat infections, and believed to stop or slow tumor growth.
- **Steel-Cut Oats:** A great source of protein and fiber. Lower glycemic than regular oats and gluten-free! Add some cinnamon and nuts and it's awesome!
- **Quinoa**: A grain that is high in protein and fiber, and low in the glycemic index. Takes the place of rice, or couscous. Tastes bland unless you add some healthy ingredients.
- **Sprouted Grain Bread:** High in Fiber and protein (see a few pages earlier).
- **Eggs:** One egg contains tons of nutrients, like six grams of protein and five grams of healthy fats.
- **Kale:** Just one cup of raw kale contains nearly three grams of protein, 2.5 grams of fiber (which helps manage blood sugar and makes you feel full). Contains Vitamins A, C, and K, and folate, a B vitamin that's key for brain development. Contains minerals including phosphorus, calcium, potassium and zinc. Both kale and spinach are leafy greens which help fight off osteoporosis, heart disease, arthritis, and several types of cancer.
- **Spinach:** Spinach is loaded with vitamins, minerals, fiber, and antioxidants—ranking third behind garlic and kale. This super food is packed with heart-friendly A and C vitamins, folate, K and magnesium. Spinach contains a chemical called oxalic acid, which binds with iron and calcium and reduces the amount your body can take in of these minerals. To improve iron absorption, eat your spinach with vitamin C-rich foods such as citrus fruit.

*Note** Be sure to check the contraindications and warnings on some of these products and foods as they can interact with certain medications and are contraindicated with some medical conditions. Always check with your health practitioner.*

Sensational Spices

1) **Turmeric** – Used to help boost weight loss! This spice stalls the spread of fat tissue by inhibiting blood vessel growth in fatty tissue! Also increases brain function, mental clarity, and memory along with rosemary, sage, mint, ginger, and black pepper!

2) **Cinnamon** – Just three grams a day aids in balancing your blood sugar levels and decreasing insulin demands. It also is known to decrease your craving for sweets. One teaspoon has about as much antioxidant benefit as a half cup of blueberries!

3) **Cayenne Pepper** – Used to help suppress hunger and sustain satiety especially when combined with green tea! Also used to burn fat.

4) **Mustard Seed** – Used to boost metabolism 20 to 25% for several hours after consumption.

5) **Ginger** – Acts as a diuretic, increases gastric mobility.

6) **Black Pepper** – Boosts metabolism, helps digestion, aids in nutrient absorption.

Anti-Inflammatory Spices

Cloves were ranked as the most potent of 24 common herbs and spices found in your spice rack. The following were found to be the top 10 most potent anti-inflammatory herbs and spices:

- Turmeric
- Cloves
- Cinnamon
- Jamaican allspice
- Apple pie spice mixture
- Oregano
- Pumpkin pie spice mixture
- Marjoram
- Sage
- Thyme
- Gourmet Italian spice

Inflammation:

Inside the body, inflammation can be beneficial—or wreak havoc with your health. Inflammation can benefit you by helping your immune system defend your body against disease-causing bacteria, viruses, and other foreign invaders that would otherwise make you sick.

The harmful side of inflammation is when it occurs without cause— in other words, when your body isn't under attack from foreign invaders. When an overactive inflammatory response happens, it can become damaging. This type of chronic inflammation is linked to autoimmune diseases like arthritis, diabetes, heart disease, cancer, and Alzheimer's disease.

But the great news is that we can do something about that kind of inflammation, as research has found that diet can play an important part in reducing inflammation. Certain vitamins in particular may help control inflammatory processes in the body.

Which vitamins have the most anti-inflammatory potential? Here's what the research has to say about vitamins and food in the reduction of inflammation.

Vitamin A

Vitamin A is commonly found in whole milk, liver, and some fortified foods. Beta-carotene is a provitamin found in carrots and many colorful vegetables that can be converted to vitamin A in the body. Vitamin A is an antioxidant. That means it protects against harmful substances in your body called free radicals, which can damage DNA and lead to cancer and other diseases. Vitamin A also has anti-inflammatory effects.

The evidence:

- A lack of enough vitamin A has been linked to inflammation in the intestines, lungs, and skin.
- For some people, taking vitamin A supplements could reduce the inflammation that contributes to conditions like inflammatory bowel disease, acne, and lung disease.

Vitamin B-6

This member of the B vitamin family is plentiful in foods like beef, turkey, vegetables, and fish. Because vitamin B-6 is water-soluble, the body is constantly ridding itself of it, so you need to restock it daily through diet.

The evidence:

- Not getting enough vitamin B6 may increase the risk for heart disease. Studies have found that people who lack enough of this vitamin have high levels of C-reactive protein (CRP), a marker of inflammation that has been linked to heart disease.
- A lack of vitamin B6 can increase inflammation associated with rheumatoid arthritis, leading to more joint damage. Yet in a vicious cycle, inflammation from rheumatoid arthritis can deplete the body's vitamin B6 stores.

Taking vitamin B6 supplements daily can correct the deficiency, yet researchers say there's no conclusive evidence it will reduce inflammation too.

Vitamin C

Your body uses this vitamin, found in oranges and other citrus fruits, for a number of different purposes. Vitamin C helps to produce collagen —the building block of skin, cartilage, ligaments, and blood vessels, and it protects against harmful substances that contribute to disease. Vitamin C is an effective antioxidant and studies suggest that it has some anti-inflammatory benefits.

The evidence:

- Taking vitamin C supplements may significantly lower levels of CRP (c-reactive protein). Having lower levels of this inflammatory marker may translate into a lower risk for heart disease.

Vitamin D

The same vitamin that works with calcium to strengthen bones can also protect against inflammation. Vitamin D can be found in fish, liver, beef, egg yolks, and some fortified foods.

Vitamin D is also produced in the body when the skin is exposed to sunlight.

The evidence:

- Vitamin D deficiency has been linked to a number of inflammatory diseases, including rheumatoid arthritis, lupus, inflammatory bowel disease, and type 1 diabetes. Taking vitamin D supplements may help reduce inflammation in people with these conditions, although this hasn't been proven. It's unclear whether or not taking vitamin D supplements can prevent any of these conditions. Vitamin D deficiency may even increase levels of inflammatory markers in healthy people.
- Vitamin D supplements may also reduce the inflammation associated with age-related diseases.
- Some studies found that people with the highest vitamin D levels had a 40% lower risk of cancer than those who had the lowest level of this vitamin.

Vitamin E
Vitamin E is another antioxidant with anti-inflammatory properties. Common food sources include nuts, seeds, and green leafy vegetables.
The evidence:

- Vitamin E comes in several different forms. The alpha-tocopherol type may help prevent heart disease by slowing the release of inflammatory substances that damage the heart.
- Alpha-tocopherol also might be effective for easing lung inflammation related to allergies. However, because studies were conducted on animals, it's not yet clear whether the results will translate to humans.

Vitamin K
Vitamin K, found in green vegetables like asparagus, broccoli, kale, and spinach, is best known for its role in helping blood clot, but research is finding that it may have other benefits, too.

The evidence:

- Getting more vitamin K can reduce levels of inflammatory markers throughout the body.

The bottom line: Good health is vitally important to live the abundant life God promises. Eating well, exercising, and living well will make you healthy and fit, mind-body-soul-spirit. It will give you spring in your step and allow you to have the energy to glorify God every day of your life. God has provided the foods of the earth for a reason... enjoy them!! (Genesis 1:29-30)

Supplement Your Diet

In February of 2015, the New York State Attorney General's office accused four major retailers of selling fraudulent and potentially dangerous herbal supplements and demanded that they remove the products from their shelves. The authorities said they had conducted tests on top-selling store brands of herbal supplements at four national retailers and found that four out of five of the products did not contain any of the herbs on their labels. The tests showed that pills labeled medicinal herbs often contained little more than cheap fillers like powdered rice, asparagus, and houseplants, and in some cases substances that could be dangerous to those with allergies.

Make sure you are taking good "pharmaceutical grade" supplements! We can't get all of our nutrients from food, but don't waste your time on vitamins with fillers and binders, which we call "bedpan bullets!" Personally my energy is off the charts when I'm taking my supplements and eating right!

The bottom line: eat right and take quality supplements to get all of your essential vitamins, minerals and nutrients in!

Intermittent Fasting

I highly recommend everyone fast having nothing but water for 12-16 hours per night. This means if your last meal was 7pm at night you don't eat again until 7am the next morning at the earliest. There are many health benefits to intermittent fasting from giving your GI system a rest to weight loss. Of course you want to keep your blood sugar stabilized throughout the day so I do not recommend IF during your waking hours. When you break the fast, start with warm water and lemon, first and then add solid food.

Food and Cancer

We know we can help prevent and reverse many cancers and disease by eating a plant-based diet.

When my sister Arlene and I researched breast cancer, the link between sugar, cancer, and obesity kept popping up. That information was not in the mainstream media then, and it's not in the mainstream media now! Not only that, doctors aren't even talking to their cancer patients about eating healthy and the links to cancer. In fact, there are world-renowned cancer institutes and oncologists that have free candy available in the lobby of their hospitals and practices.

Back in 1924, Otto Warburg, PhD, a Nobel Prize–winning biochemist, proposed the hypothesis that cancer is a metabolic disease that affects the way cells use food to make energy. Warburg believed that cancer cells exhibit a preference for using sugar to fuel themselves, even when the oxygen for normal cellular processes were available. He wrote: "Cancer, above all other diseases, has countless secondary causes. But even for cancer, there is only one prime cause. Summarized in a few words, the prime cause of cancer is the replacement of the respiration of oxygen in normal cells by a fermentation of sugar."

Unfortunately, the general direction of cancer research over the past 40 years has been biased toward genetic causes with drug-based treatments, and little progress has been made toward a cure, leaving many patients with a dismal future and death.

Recently, though, Dr. Thomas Seyfried has backed Warburg's work in his book *Cancer as a Metabolic Disease: On the Origin Management and Prevention of Cancer.* Dr. Seyfried argues that cancer is not a genetic disease but a metabolic disease. Metabolic diseases are conditions in which the metabolism, or the making of energy from the food we eat, is abnormal or dysfunctional in some way. Normal cells are able to efficiently use the food we eat and the oxygen we inhale to complete normal cellular respiration and make adenosine triphosphate (ATP), our cellular energy source.

The second type of cellular fuel is ketone bodies, which come from fatty acids. They come from fats we eat or the metabolism of fats. This fat metabolism process is called ketogenesis, and the shift in metabolism that favors fats as the primary fuel for energy is called ketosis. Long story short, cancer cells can't use ketones, and must have glucose to stay alive and grow. In very simple terms, a high-carbohydrate diet has been found to feed cancer cells, and a low-carbohydrate diet has been found to starve cancer cells. Remember it's not just the sugar we're talking about, it is the foods that turn into sugar as well. There is so much research out there about spontaneous regression of tumor cells based on lifestyle and food changes, without any chemotherapy medication. Again, it's not reported in the mainstream media, but the facts are there when you begin to research.

I am asked quite often by my clients what I would do if I had cancer. Am I against chemotherapy treatment for cancer? I won't answer that, because I believe it's an individual personal decision that people need to make for themselves. But I can tell you this: what we eat matters. It can either feed most cancers and diseases or prevent it, so why wouldn't we use food as the main part of our treatment plans for patients? Why do doctors and our health care system avoid that component of the treatment plan? Why do we have to fight with our insurance companies to pay for a nutrition or healthy eating program, but they will pay for diagnostic tests, co-pays, surgeries, medications, lap band surgeries for weight loss and the like?

I look at sweets as carcinogens, and I am no longer tempted to eat them, nor am I addicted to them. If I want to taste something I do, but it's not something I crave or have to have like it was when sweets once controlled my life! There was a time that I lived to eat desserts! But I broke the chain... not by my own strength, but through Christ alone (and the help of a detox)! I am free!! Now you have to break the chain!

Cancer-Fighting Foods:

Phytochemicals in shiitake mushrooms block the enzyme aromatase from producing estrogen. Controlling aromatase activity can help decrease estrogen levels, which controls and kills hormone-dependent breast cancers. In addition, mushrooms also demonstrate the ability to inhibit cancer cell activity and slow tumor growth in all areas.

Other anti-cancer foods and drinks include:

- Pomegranates
- Cinnamon
- Turmeric
- Blueberries
- Mushrooms
- Grapes
- Green tea
- Vitamin C

The Raw Truth for Optimum Health:

- Eat mostly a plant-based diet with at least 80% vegetables, and 20% or less of fruit.
- Avoid all processed food. And if it's white, don't bite.
- Drink mostly what you are made of: water.
- Avoid bad fats (trans, saturated). Eat good fat.
- Eat only organic animal products, and only organic non-GMO fruits and vegetables.
- Exercise most days of the week for thirty to sixty minutes.
- Get seven to eight hours of sleep.
- Manage stress.
- Don't worry. Philippians 4:6 it! Let go, let God.

7 Food Raw Truths:

1. Just because you are absent from disease does not mean you are well.
2. Eating right and exercising are a decision and a choice. Overeating is usually because of a heart issue, not a food issue. Don't let any food or drink become your God. Eat and drink only for the glory of God. Self-control is a fruit of the Spirit.
3. Remember our gut microbiome is essential to our over-all health from your physical health to your mental health.
4. You will eat what you crave, and crave what you eat.

107

5. Eat food, not food-like things. Eat the food of the earth that God created, and that's what you will crave.
6. If it comes from a plant, eat it; if it was made in a plant, don't eat it! Yes, it's a little more expensive to eat organic, but you will spend the time and the money either way.
7. You will either spend the time and the money treating disease with doctors' appointments, tests, treatments, and co-pays, or you will spend the time and the money preventing disease by eating right and exercising. Which is better for you?

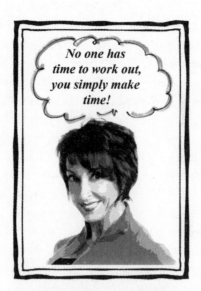

No one has time to work out, you simply make time!

TRUTH FOUR
Fitness Is For Life

MY MOM ALWAYS said, "Robbie, if you don't take care of yourself you can't take care of your family." For the most part, she was referring to making sure I ate, but she also encouraged me to exercise and even joined the gym with me when she was younger! I knew if I didn't take care of myself, I wouldn't be able to take care of my children or Mom, so I never felt guilty about making the time or spending the money to eat right and go the gym.

Here's the thing: you can be healthy and not be fit, or you can be fit and not healthy. In other words, you can eat right and not exercise and be unhealthy, or you can exercise and not eat right and be unhealthy. You can't out-exercise a bad diet! It just doesn't work.

First, you really do have to cut the excuses and make time for exercise in your life, the same way you have to make the time to brush your teeth, do your bills, clean your house, cut up your veggies, prepare your food and deliberately eat right. But when it comes to exercise and eating right, you have to do it as if your life depends on it, because in so many ways it does.

In my thirty-plus years in the industry, I have heard every excuse in the book why people can't find the time to exercise. And truly most of the excuses I've heard aren't valid. We all have the same amount of hours in a day. Get up earlier, go to bed later, exercise in your lunch hour and find the time at least three days a week and preferably seven for at least 30 minutes! People who have an excuse not to exercise when it's cold out will find an excuse not to exercise when it's hot out. They will find an excuse if they aren't committed no matter what.

Now if you haven't exercised in a while, you can start slowly. You should set up your life so that you are nudged into exercising every day naturally. By that I mean don't take the closest parking space at work or at the gym, so you'll have to walk farther. Take the stairs instead of taking the elevator. Do things that require you to move naturally. Although moving naturally doesn't replace getting your cardio and resistive training in at the gym, it does benefit you to move more during the day.

Exercise has been part of my life for the last thirty-plus years. That's certainly not because I have a lot of time on my hands, or because I love hard work, or because I love to sweat and breathe heavy. It's not because I love pushing myself harder and farther every day (although sometimes that's true), and it's not because it's convenient, it's easy, or it's something I don't need to be deliberate about. The truth is:

- I can always think of something else I can do (my to-do list keeps growing).
- I don't always feel like pushing myself (sometimes I'm just tired).
- It's not always convenient for me to work out (I have to go outside, face the cold and drive to the gym).
- It's not easy (nothing good in life is easy).

I have to be very deliberate about working out if it's going to happen. I have, however, always been driven to feel great and be healthy because as a nurse I have seen the sad results of those who haven't taken care of themselves— and that impacted me very early on.

I tell my clients, "Just show up at the gym. We'll take care of you once you get there." Getting there, or starting to exercise (at home, outside, etc.) is the hardest part. But once you actually get there and start, you'll feel so much better! I truly believe Nike was talking about this issue when they said, "Just do it."

By the way, this doesn't mean you have to do an hour of kickboxing (although that would be fantastic)! Do whatever you can do. If all you have time for is a twenty-minute run, then do a twenty-minute run. If all your health allows you to do is take a walk or ride a stationary bike, then get out there and go for a walk or ride that bike!

The only time failure creeps in is when you don't try. Just start!

Think about this—just thirty minutes of exercise a day can give you the following benefits and more:

- Boosts your immune system and wards off illness.
- Reduces your risk of coronary heart disease, some cancers, diabetes, high blood pressure, and high cholesterol.
- Helps maintain healthy bones and muscles.
- Helps control joint swelling and pain associated with arthritis.
- Helps reduce body fat.
- Improves body composition (more muscle, less fat).

That thirty minutes also reduces symptoms of anxiety and depression and boosts your mood. Exercise increases your stamina and reduces fatigue (energy produces energy). If you're trying to lose weight, exercise is your best friend, because exercise builds muscle and muscle dictates metabolism. And let's face it—working out helps you look gr8 and feel gr8!

The Benefits of Exercise Are:

- You will feel and become healthier and fit.
- You will look like you exercise, which builds self-confidence.
- You will be more comfortable with your body.
- You will reach your goals.
- You will be more productive.
- You will be more disciplined, which will infiltrate into other areas of your life.

So you still think you don't have time to exercise? I have been working in a gym for more than thirty years, surrounded by sweaty bodies, and I don't have time to exercise either! I can tell you this: nobody has time to work out or prepare his or her healthy foods for the day or week. You just have to make time, because it's that important.

We all have the same twenty-four hours in a day. Your allotment of time is no different than mine, but what you do with that time makes all the difference in the quality of your life, the length of your life, your body composition, your energy level, and your level of fitness.

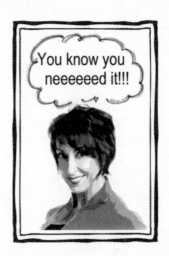

Excuses Are Just Excuses. Cut them out!

Have you ever tried any of these crazy excuses for not exercising? I've heard them all:

- I can't exercise; when I was a kid I had a lazy eye, and it spread to the rest of my body.
- Situps will build muscle and make my stomach bigger.
- Swimming won't help me lose weight—look at whales!
- I am in shape already. I'm round, and round is a shape!
- I listen to my doctor, and he/she doesn't tell me to lose weight or exercise, so it must not be important!
- I get enough exercise cleaning my house!
- I have no time… (la la la la la…)
- Your heart is only good for so many beats, and that's it! Don't waste them on exercise!

- Speeding up your heart will not make you live longer. That's like saying you can extend the life of your car by driving it faster.
- Want to live longer? Take a nap. That's what I do.
- I eat, and I don't exercise, and I'm not fat...

Not to be judgmental or rude, but when someone tells me they don't have thirty minutes in their day to work out, I just want to say "Yeah, whatever!" Did you go on Facebook today? Did you sit in front of the TV today? Did you read a book or the newspaper? Did you try to get up early or stay up late to make exercise happen? Did you get a lunch break? Are there ten minutes in your morning, afternoon or evening that you can carve out to equal thirty minutes?

You really do have to look at your day (the night before) and plan out thirty minutes or a one-hour block to work out, or I am here to tell you it's not going to happen! You have to put it in your calendar, in your phone, in your daytimer, on the refrigerator calendar, just like a doctor's appointment. You can probably eliminate a couple of those doctor's appointments if you make time to actually prevent disease rather than just treat disease.

Are you too tired to work out?

Many times people are too tired because they have not exercised. Energy produces energy, and you will have more energy after you work out! Trust me on this! If you are one of those people that has a hard time getting motivated on your own, I urge you to take a group exercise class. In group exercise classes, even if you don't feel like working out, energy produces energy, and it starts bouncing between people and off the walls. Before you know it, sixty minutes goes by, and you're drenched in sweat!

Here's an important point: throughout my career, I have seen over and over people who focus on eating right without the exercise, who don't get results. And vice versa! There are those people who think they can eat whatever they want and not exercise and be lean and fit. Negative on both accounts. You really do need both—eating right *and* exercising are the keys to a healthy and fit life. There are no sweatless quickies. You will be a much better mother, wife, husband, father, friend, or employee if you are healthy, happy, and energetic. You owe it to yourself and to your family to be healthy. When a person in the family is sick, it affects everyone, and the reverse is true. Exercise can prevent and help reverse disease.

It is a privilege and opportunity to reap the blessings of good health. Look at exercise as something you "get" to do, not something you "have" to do.

There Are Five Components of Physical Fitness and Health

1. Cardiovascular exercise
2. Muscular strength
3. Muscular endurance
4. Flexibility
5. Body composition

Exercise Recommendations:

Always check with your doctor before beginning any new exercise program. Here are some guidelines and goals to aim for:

- Moderate to intense cardio, thirty to sixty minutes a day, three to seven days a week. Build up to this gradually.
- Strength-training exercises, thirty to sixty minutes a day, three days per week.
- The Fit Principle – Stands for Frequency Intensity Time and Type. You can manipulate the FIT principle to reach your goals. In other words, if you won't have 7 days a week to work out for 30 minutes, then work out 3-4 days per week and make it longer and harder.
- The Overload Principle – Meaning you have to push yourself a little farther, a little harder to reach the training effect as adaptation takes place.

Too tired to work out? Remember energy produces energy. Persevere…

Cardiovascular Exercise

If your time is limited, aerobic activity should be your exercise of choice due to the overall health benefits:

- Burning fat
- Utilizing calories
- Improving your cardiovascular system

114

- Sweating toxins out of your body
- Increasing your energy
- Reducing your stress
- Decreasing the aging process
- Getting an endorphin high

How Much Cardio Do You Need?

The American College of Sports Medicine and the American Heart Association recommend thirty to sixty minutes of moderate to vigorous intensity activity on most days of the week. But, the truth is, everyone's cardio needs differ and depend on factors such as:

- How many calories you take in (although it's not just about calories in and calories out)
- How hard you exercise
- Your metabolism, age and gender
- Your fitness level
- Your body fat percentage and weight
- Your exercise schedule
- What your goal is (lose weight, gain weight, burn fat, get a stronger cardiovascular system, stay young, increase energy, etc.)

Pumping Iron

It's a fact: weight training is the best way to crank up your resting metabolic rate. As you get older, you lose muscle and your resting metabolic rate drops, but weight training can rev it right back up again. A pound of muscle burns up to nine times the calories a pound of fat does. In fact, a woman who weighs 130 pounds and is muscular burns more calories than a sedentary 120-pound woman of the same height. Regular strength training can increase your resting metabolic rate anywhere from 6.8 to 7.8 percent. (That

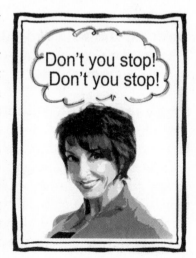

means that if you weigh 120 pounds, you could burn around 100 more calories a day, even when you're just watching TV.)

Bonus: Weight training also gives your metabolism a short-term boost. When women lift weights, their metabolisms remain in overdrive for up to two hours after the last bench press, allowing them to burn as many as 100 extra calories, according to a study published in *Medicine and Science in Sports and Exercise.*

Revving Up Your Workouts

Adding interval training—bursts of high-intensity moves combined with lower intensity and/or strength training—to your workout is a great metabolism booster. Studies have shown that people who do interval training twice a week [in addition to cardio] lose twice as much weight as those who do just a regular cardio workout. One of my exercise videos is called "Raw NRG Extreme Interval Training," where I lead you through four to five–minute intervals of cardio and weight lifting! Talk about kicking butt! It's the best workout for body shaping!

You can easily incorporate interval training into your workout by inserting a thirty-second sprint into your jog every five minutes, or by adding a one-minute incline walk to your treadmill workout. Since your body is working harder, it's a more intense workout, and you therefore burn more calories.

Working Out with Weights

Here are some common questions and answers I often get asked about working out with weights.

How heavy do the weights have to be?

This differs for everyone. Begin by choosing both heavy and lighter weights. Heavy weights are used for the larger muscle groups like back, chest, legs and glutes, and lighter weights are used for the smaller muscle groups like biceps, deltoids, and triceps. Use a weight that provides enough resistance to make it tough to push out those last few reps (the number of times you lift the weight) while still allowing you to maintain proper form. If the weight is easy to lift after the fourth rep, then the weight is too light. If you're struggling early, it's too heavy. Keep in mind you'll probably use a variety of weights throughout your workout.

How many exercises/reps should I be doing?

The American College of Sports Medicine (ACSM) recommends individuals perform eight to ten strength-training exercises each session. Aim to target each major muscle group including arms, chest, back, abs, and legs. Complete eight to twelve reps of each exercise to improve your overall strength, boost your metabolism, and sculpt those muscles. Perform two to three sets per exercise or do four-minute intervals per muscle group combined with rest.

If my time is limited, what should I do?

If your time is limited, aerobic activity should be your exercise choice due to the overall health benefits. With that said, cardio is not going to shape your body but strength training will, so you need both. My preference is interval training, which is a combination of both cardio and body-sculpting with weights. I am not big on weights with cardio, as too many people end up swinging the weights and putting stress on their joints.

> *In his heart a man plans his course, but the Lord determines his steps. (Proverbs 16:9)*

We just need to pray for God's will and stop trying to be the commander in chief! Let His will be done.

> *Consider it pure joy, my brothers, whenever you face trials of many kinds, because you know that the testing of your faith develops **perseverance**. Perseverance must finish its work so that you may be mature and complete, not lacking anything. (James 1:2-4)*

Important Facts

• Exercise your body, mind, soul, and spirit as if your life depends on it—because it does.

- You can exercise all day long, but if your dietary habits aren't promoting health and wellness, you will be thick and tired.
- Although exercise is important, 90% of our body composition has to do with our dietary habits, not how much we exercise.
- Awesome abs are made in the kitchen!

When you work out, remember to thank God for your healthy body. So many people can't even walk through the front door of the gym alone, let alone work out. I don't know about you, but that's another thing that motivates me.

With that said, here are some tips for setting up an effective cardio program:

- If you're a beginner, start with three days of the cardio exercise of your choice, working at a level you can handle, for a minimum of ten to twenty minutes.
- Add time each week to work your way up to thirty to forty-five minutes of continuous exercise.
- As you get stronger, try interval training once a week to help boost endurance and burn more calories, where you do intervals of high intensity combined with periods of low intensity or strength.
- Work your way up to four to six days of cardio and try to vary what you do and how hard you work (go harder on the days you have more energy and push the days you don't).
- And don't forget the weights!

When I don't work out or eat right, I feel sluggish, irritable, fat, cranky, and tired, and I don't want to get up in the morning or face the day. My body is just telling me something is wrong! It's funny because when you feel like that all the time, and you never experience how good it feels to eat right and work out—you don't really know what you're missing!

In fact you don't know how bad you feel until you start feeling good!

I can't go more than two days without working out, or I start to feel really awful.

Now, do I love running? Not necessarily— but I love being outside and getting the best bang for my buck. I love how running makes my legs feel, and I love pushing my body to the max, feeling my heart pump hard, and feeling that endorphin high. So lace up your sneakers, or tune up your bikes, and get out there.

Just like everything else, the hardest part is just starting. So block the time out, gear up your iPod, and put one foot in front of the other and take it to the streets. Trust me: you will feel so much better afterwards! And whatever it is that you did not do to make time for your workout, you can do that thing much better after you work out!

The health benefits of just thirty minutes of physical activity a day are immense. It:

- Reduces the risk of dying from coronary heart disease and developing high blood pressure, colon cancer, and diabetes.
- Helps maintain healthy bones and muscles.
- Helps control joint swelling and pain associated with arthritis.
- Can help reduce blood pressure in some women with hypertension.
- Helps maintain a healthy heart by keeping your arteries clear, increasing the concentration of "good" cholesterol and decreasing the concentration of "bad" cholesterol in your blood.
- Boosts your mood, possibly easing depression and reduces the tension associated with anxiety.
- Promotes relaxation.
- Increases your stamina and reduces fatigue.
- Improves body composition by burning fat and utilizing calories.
- Decreases symptoms of PMS and menopause in women.
- Wards off viral illnesses by activating your immune system.

Your Brain

Your brain loves oxygen. The more you exercise, the more oxygen reaches your brain, and the better your mental state. Exercise is the one and only thing that will increase your mental alertness, improve your memory, and give you stability and tranquility with no side effects! Get moving!

Before You Start Exercising

Before you get started, you need to know your numbers. You can't manage what you don't measure!

Take the following measurements the day before you start the program and record them on your phone or journal.

1) Your weight – Weigh yourself first thing in the morning without clothes on.
2) Your height – in feet and inches.
3) Your waist – Using a tape measure, find the widest point around your belly button, not where your belt is. Use your belly button as the guide.
4) Your hips – Using a tape measure, find the widest point around your hips.
5) Your thigh circumference – Stand up straight with your hand and fingers on your thighs. Put the tape measure at the tip of the third finger around your thigh.
6) Your body fat percent. Buy a device or stop in the gym and ask someone to take the measurements for you.

It's so much more than just about the scale and numbers, it's about your health! Losing weight does not automatically mean you are losing excess body fat. You could be losing muscle density that your body needs to function properly, prevent disease and reduce health risks. This will slow down your metabolic rate. Many people who do too much cardio and not enough weight lifting are in the category. You also could be skinny but fat, look thin but still have the same health risks an obese person has.

Body weight includes body fat, bones, blood, muscles, and water. Body fat percentage refers to the amount of body fat mass that's a part of the total body weight.

Body fat measurements are very important because excess fat increases your risk of heart disease, diabetes, some cancers to name a few. Body fat stats do not move a lot like the scale or inches do. A little change in body fat % up or down means a lot in terms of your health (and how you lean you look). And if you're going to work out you might as well look like you work out with body fat loss and muscle growth (definition). That comes with working out with weights, eating right, and doing cardio.

You can use a bioelectrical impedance (BI) method to determine body fat percent by a small electric conductivity. Your weight, age, height, and gender are programmed into the machine and you hold the machine in your hands.

Body fat consists of essential body fat and storage fat. Essential body fat is present in the nerve tissues, bone marrow, and organs (all membranes), and we cannot lose this fat without compromising physiological function.

Storage fat, on the other hand, represents an energy reserve that accumulates when excess energy is ingested and decreases when more energy is expended than consumed.

Essential body fat is approximately 2-4% of body mass for men and 10-12% of body mass for women (referenced through The American Council on Exercise). Women are believed to have more essential body fat than men because of childbearing and hormonal functions.

Body Fat Percentages

- Athlete levels are considered 6–13% for men and 14–20% for women.
- Fitness levels are considered 14–17% for men and 21–24% for women.
- Acceptable ranges are 18–25% for men and 25–31% for women.

Obese levels are 26%+ for men and 32%+ for women. Many experts consider 25% for men and 30% for women obese.

In general, an average total body fat percentage (essential plus storage fat) is between 12% and 15% for young men and between 25% and 28% for young women, but it depends on your age greatly.

While BMI largely increases as adiposity increases, due to differences in body composition, other indicators of body fat give more accurate results; for example, individuals with greater muscle mass or larger bones will have higher BMIs inaccurately showing up as obese.

It's based on height and weight only. The BMI assumes a normal muscle distribution so people who work out or athletes with a lot of muscle mass need to take the measurements with a grain of salt since it doesn't take high muscle percent or low body fat percent into account.

Regardless of gender, or age, a "healthy weight" reading for BMI falls between 18.5 and 24.9. A BMI of 25 or higher is considered overweight and anything over 29.9 is considered obese. This does not take into consideration the amount of muscle mass a person has. Again—I don't use this at all for that reason. I recommend measurements of body fat percentage, diet history, exercise patterns, and family history.

BMI also does not take into account age, gender, or muscle mass. Nor does it distinguish between lean body mass and fat mass. As a result, some people, such as heavily muscled athletes, may have a high BMI even though they don't have a high percentage of body fat. In others, such as elderly people, BMI may appear normal even though muscle has been lost with aging.

It makes no allowance for the relative proportions of bone, muscle and fat in the body. But bone is denser than muscle and twice as dense as fat, so a person with strong bones, good muscle tone and low fat will have a high BMI. Thus, athletes and fit, health-conscious people who work out a lot tend to find themselves classified as overweight or even obese.

The CDC says on its website "the BMI is a reliable indicator of body fatness for people." I highly disagree.

I was one of those people years ago who weighed myself 10 times a day. When I finally realized it was more about my health and not about the numbers, and that how I fit into the normal "weight range chart" didn't matter, I was able to focus on my health and really "let go, to let God." I actually started focusing on the things that mattered—like having the energy to work towards what God's purpose was in my life. I started thinking about how I need my health and energy to do what God is calling me to do.

I believe in the principles I teach, and I'm convicted. But it never escapes my mind that although my platform is health and fitness, my motivation, focus, mission, passion, strength is for God and from God. Again, I know I need to be healthy to live out God's plan for my life.

We are on our way to an abundant life, to serve God with more energy, health and passion than we ever imagined we could have. This is a journey, not a race, and God is the compass. All we need to do is follow Him and He will direct our paths....

Record The Following Measurements Monthly:

- Weight on a scale, no shoes
- Height
- Thigh circumference with a tape measure at the widest part of your thigh
- Waist size with a tape measure around at your belly button
- Hip size with a tape measure at the widest part of your hip
- Body fat percent (you may need to stop in a gym or have a health coach/practitioner do this for you)
- Blood pressure again done by a doctor, health coach or practitioner

You should monitor and record your weights and measures at the beginning of every month.

Dust off your home gym stuff, or renew your health club membership! Consider purchasing a personal fitness tracker like Jawbone or FitBit. There are ton of phone apps as well.

> *Since we have these promises, dear friends, let us purify ourselves from everything that contaminates the body and spirit, perfecting holiness out of reverence for God. (2 Corinthians 7:1)*

Plateaus

A plateau in the health and fitness arena usually means that the scale is not moving. It's very common for our bodies to hit a plateau where we are pushing hard, working out, eating right, yet nothing seems to be changing in our bodies. The scale is the same, or maybe you even gained weight, your clothes are still tight or maybe they seem tighter than before! This is the time where you evaluate and perhaps even change what you are doing.

There are five things you can do to push through a body plateau.

1) Journal what you are eating and drinking every day. You should also write down how you FEEL, not just what you are doing. People who journal about their food, their finances, their relationships etc. are 50% more successful than people who don't. When you know you have to write it down, and you take a look at it afterwards,

it's eye-opening at times. Most of my clients don't realize how often they lick the spoon, or eat their kid's leftovers until they start journaling. When you are having a great day, you can look back and see what made it a great day. When you don't have energy or you backslide, you can look at that and see why to help prevent it from happening again. Research all shows that Journaling is an integral part in changing lifestyle habits.

2) Start exercising, or if you are already exercising, pick up the intensity, frequency, duration, or type of exercise. Take it to a higher level. Don't go to the gym and lift the same amount of weights each day, or put the same amount of intensity into your cardio routine. Push yourself to increase your workload thereby working on the overload principle (when you push yourself past your comfort zone) to get greater results.

3) Cut out the sugar, junk food, white stuff, dairy, and processed food if you haven't done so already. This stuff will sabotage any results you are trying to get. You can work out at the gym four hours a day but if you are still putting junk in, you are going to feel awful, risk your health, and gain weight. You can't out-exercise a bad diet!

4) Cut out the grains for a short time. You may have a gluten or wheat sensitivity, which is preventing you from losing weight. By omitting grains from your diet for at least two weeks and then adding them back gradually you can see if you are sensitive. You may experience bloating, you may crave sugar, and you may even gain weight. These are all fairly good signs that you may be wheat or gluten sensitive.

5) When all else fails—detox. And it's always better to do one under a health professional's care where you can take it to a higher level of detox.

Trying the above tips will help you push past a plateau. The only time failure creeps in completely is when you don't try.

To your health and body composition, these 7 things remain true:

1) Portions matter
2) The type of food you eat matters
3) Exercise matters
4) Who you hang out with matters (hang out with like-minded people who also want to be healthy)
5) Managing stress and sleep matters
6) Drinking enough water matters
7) Journaling matters

Remember you eat what you crave and you crave what you eat!

You are on your way to an abundant life, to serve God with more energy, health and passion than you ever imagined you could have. This is a journey, not a race, and God is the compass. All we need to do is follow Him, and He will direct our paths.

Robbie's Survival Tips

- Don't go for seconds
- Leave space between your food on your plate
- Eat healthy before a party or BYO (bring your own)
- Master healthy mini-snacks to keep your blood sugar stable and keep your metabolism and energy elevated
- Drink sixty-four ounces of water per day minimum
- Prepare meals and snacks ahead of time
- Make veggies the main dish
- Eat whole grains
- Drink a glass of water before eating. Cuts your intake down 20%
- Look for low net carbs (Carbs minus sugar alcohol minus fiber)
- Include lean sources of protein, three to six ounces per meal
- Get enough sleep
- Don't skip meals (especially breakfast)
- Exercise
- Incorporate twenty-five grams of fiber per day (at least five grams per item)

- Look for no more than five grams of sugar (and make sure the ingredients are healthy) and stay in single digit net carbs.
- Journal – remember people who do are 50% more successful than those you don't.
- Read labels – look at ingredients first, then carbs, then sugar, protein, fat, and fiber.
- Green tea helps boost your immune system, reduces the risk of osteoporosis and breast cancer, and is a natural fat burner. It contains the antioxidant power of red wine.

Raw Truth Tips For Exercising:

- Always exercise on Monday to kick start the week. Research shows that people who exercise regularly are healthier, have more energy, think more clearly, sleep better, are more productive, look great, feel great, and have a later onset of dementia. Why wait until Tuesday? Kick-start your week and get a schedule down.
- Exercise at whatever time works in your schedule. It doesn't matter if it's early morning, lunchtime, or nighttime. What matters is that you do it.
- Try not to skip exercising two days in a row and if you do get right back to it. Two days turns into four days, turns into a week, turns into a month, and pretty soon you forgot that you ever exercised to begin with. Be consistent and build exercise time into your daily plans.
- Give yourself credit for doing anything. If it's twenty minutes, thirty minutes or sixty, high intensity, moderate intensity, low intensity—at least you did something! You are not always going to feel energetic every day. On the days you feel a lot of energy, hit it hard. On the days you don't have the energy, work out anyway but cut yourself some slack. Chances are you will find energy through working out!
- Work out most days of the week. Build it into your schedule and just do it no matter what.
- Forget the excuses. I've heard them all and none of them are more important than your health and being able to be there for your kids and/or family with a beating heart and breath in your lungs. My

126

mom always told me that if I didn't take care of myself, I wouldn't be able to take care of anyone else. It's kind of like "put your oxygen mask on first and then assist your child" mentality. My mom also told me "When the Mom goes down, the ship goes down." That's enough for me to get motivated!

- Get a Fit Bit or wearable technology to measure your workouts. You can't manage what you don't measure and it will keep you motivated!

- I know so many people that keep paying their gym memberships year after year and never go. Having a gym membership does not mean you are going to get in shape and healthy any more than standing in your garage makes you a car. It takes showing up at the gym and exercising, or working out at home, and it takes good dietary habits as well. But you know that, right? So just do it!

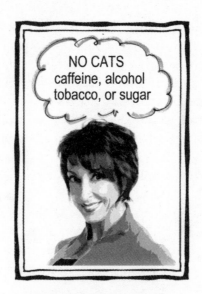

TRUTH FIVE
Detox For Health

IN THE UNITED States and Canada, we are getting fatter and more unhealthy. Clearly, what we are doing isn't working. The last thirty years of diets didn't work, and it's because "calories in and calories out" isn't the only answer. If it were about calories in and calories out, then everyone killing themselves in the gym would be lean and mean!

What worked in terms of your diet and exercise program in your twenties and thirties doesn't work in your forties, fifties and beyond. You need to tweak them as you age in order to stay ahead of the curve! Every decade that goes by causes you to lose muscle mass, which in turn slows down your metabolism. But I'm here to tell you, that doesn't need to be the case! Muscle is key to sculpting your body and also to turning your body into a fat-burning machine!

The benefits of eating right go beyond weight loss as you all know, but I know people are always concerned about losing weight. With that said, I could nail these seven things to the wall when it comes to success with fat loss, weight loss, and health:

1. You need to reset your metabolism and rid the toxins with a detox.
2. You need to eat clean and know what that means.
3. You need to exercise most days of the week.
4. You need good gut health.
5. You need proper hormone regulation.
6. You need to manage your stress and sleep.
7. You need to monitor your numbers (refer to the Exercise section on how to measure your body).
8. And remember God's Word says,

Whether you eat or drink or whatever you do, do it all to the glory of God. (1 Corinthians 10:31)

The mainstream definition of "eating healthy or clean" is completely wrong from what eating healthy and clean should be. That word, "healthy" means something different to everyone, and I see that every time I ask people to write down what they consider their healthy eating plan for three to five days.

The Raw Truth is, if you are cutting or counting calories, counting points, avoiding fat, eating "heart-healthy" vegetable oils, having bread for every meal, think wheat bread is healthy, or just eating salads, you've been terribly misled.

Without knowing each and every one of you, I know this: Many problems stem from yo-yo dieting, which is losing and gaining significant amounts of weight over and over again, which messes with your system. Crash dieting or starving yourself slows down your metabolic rate to a snail's pace.

And eating high-glycemic foods and processed junk food will cause you to crave more of the same and cause your body to store fat. And did you know that sleep deprivation and stress causes weight gain? More on those topics in later chapters!

The good thing is, there is hope for people who have been experiencing any of these issues if they focus on exercise, overcome the obstacles, learn what triggers bad behavior, practice behavior modification, and eat nutrient-dense foods which fuel the body and keep metabolism high to burn fat and utilize calories.

The best fuel for your body is very clean, highly nutrient-dense food, which is food from the earth that God created. The one you don't need to read a label on. Eating well isn't about high carbs, low carbs, or no carbs; it's about focusing on the right carbs. It's not about high-fat, low-fat or no-fat; it's about the right fat. It's not cutting out grains forever; it's about eating nutrient-dense grains like sprouted grains. It's not about a 12-week program or a year of dieting; it's about learning and eating well the rest of your life. It's not about being deprived of guilty pleasures; it's about having your cake and eating it too with "no-guilt goodies" that are made with healthy ingredients.

The amino acids we derive from protein are used to make neurotransmitters (brain chemicals) that actually can help control appetite, reduce cravings, and balance mood swings. The best way to overcome those cravings is to detox, as we will talk about later. But you also want to have a good source of protein and fiber with every meal to keep your blood sugar stabilized. Have three balanced meals a day that include protein and fiber at regular intervals throughout the day (or, if you're like me, you may have four or five smaller meals). A balanced meal contains nutrient-dense foods including good sources of protein, good fat, and the right carbohydrates.

You drop weight drastically when you eliminate wheat and other gluten-containing grains from your diet (like barley and rye). The key is to control and manage the amount of carbohydrates and sugars in your diet to your own individual tolerance levels in an effort to stabilize your blood sugars and help you lose weight. This is where bio-individuality once again comes in.

Eliminating wheat and gluten products— even the so-called healthy whole grain wheat— from our diets, I believe, is the key to permanent weight loss and can offer relief from a broad spectrum of health and digestive problems.

Why Detox?

When I suggest a detox to my clients, most of the time they have a look on their face that looks like I asked them to avoid food for a week! A detox doesn't mean you are going to be starving yourself, or eating weird-looking food from the sea that you can't pronounce. Or that you won't be able to go to work or function because you will be flat out in bed. None of these are true!

Anyone who wants to feel great and look great should do a medically sound detox!

During the Raw Truth Recharge detox that I recommend, we will get rid of the sugar and caffeine that causes our blood sugar to increase, causes disease and sickness, increases our cravings for sweets, and sabotages our desire to lose weight. We are also getting rid of the carcinogens, processed foods, pesticides, hydrogenated oils, toxins, dairy, food colorings, nitrates, steroids, and chemicals that wreak havoc on our metabolism and health.

A detox is really paramount to cut the cravings for sweets. And as I've mentioned, cancer has a sweet tooth. That in and of itself is enough for me to turn away from sugar, that poison that is as addictive as a drug.

Within just a few days of a detox, you will see that your skin will clear up, your joints won't hurt anymore, your brain will think more clearly, your digestion will improve, your breathing will improve, you will sleep better, get up easier, you will have more energy, and your clothes will be looser! I have had clients stop using a cane and a wheelchair that they previously needed, and these are people who thought I was crazy when I said they could get healthy and ditch those pieces of equipment. Clients who couldn't even walk because of pain are actually working out at the end of detox!

When you cut out the junk, processed food, simple carbs, etc., you can expect to lose anywhere from five to ten pounds during a two-week detox. You will lose inches in your waist, hips, and thighs, you will increase your energy, decrease your body fat and weight, stabilize your blood sugar, and more! All of these positive results will happen in just a few days! Did you hear that? In days!

The first few days of getting off sugar and caffeine will be a little uncomfortable. Now, this doesn't mean you can't work or that you will be in the bathroom all the time. It just means you will get headaches and feel irritable. But you can handle that in order to feel better in the long run, right?

Always consult a board-certified expert in the field, and frankly, that's probably not someone who considers themselves a fitness person who self-learns, and it may or may not mean your doctor depending on his training and expertise! Doctors and health practitioners should be versed in preventing disease and helping their patients be motivated and educated to lose weight and exercise, but that is not always the case. They need to be walking the talk as well! When I'm looking for a dentist, I don't go to one who has bad teeth. Get the point?

The first step to eating healthy, being healthy, losing weight, cutting cravings, jump-starting your metabolism, clearing up your skin, or increasing your energy is committing to a medically sound detox to reset your metabolism and clean out your digestive system. You can eat all the best clean food in the world, but unless your metabolism, digestive system and other organs are operating optimally, you will never see the results you're striving for. I have seen this over and over for many years working in the gym. People are eating right and exercising but still not getting results! You need to reset and jump-start your metabolism, like you reset your computer or phone by turning it off and back on.

God's Word tells us:

> *Since we have these promises, dear friends, let us purify ourselves from everything that contaminates body and spirit, perfecting holiness out of reverence for God. (2 Corinthians 7:1)*

> *Do not be wise in your own eyes; fear the Lord and shun evil. This will bring health to your body and nourishment to your bones. (Proverbs 3:7-8)*

To help your metabolism operate efficiently and give you energy and a lean body, your body has mechanisms to rid itself of harmful toxins and substances, which come from our food, alcohol, and medications. These create a trap, and even if you start eating right, the nutrients have trouble being absorbed, and you probably won't lose weight without doing a detox. This will lead to bloating, inflammation, overeating, cravings, and yo-yo dieting. It's like putting oil in your car and never changing the filter. Your car wouldn't operate on all cylinders, and neither will your body!

Fresh fruits and vegetables contain the phytonutrients I talked about earlier, and living enzymes that cleanse the digestive tract and keep it functioning optimally. Phytonutrients are plant-derived nutrients that contain antioxidants. Antioxidants are natural compounds that protect the body from harmful free radicals. A free radical is an atom or group of atoms that cause damage to cells, impairing the immune system, leading to infection and various diseases such as heart disease and cancer; therefore, antioxidants play a beneficial role in the prevention of disease. Scientists also believe free radicals to be the basis of the aging process. Enzymes are proteins that initiate and speed up the rate at which changes and chemical reactions take place in your body. They also help cells to communicate with one another. Without enzymes, the chemical reactions would take place too slowly to keep you alive.

I recommend that people detox seasonally. A detox can mean something different to everyone. Bio-individuality is important; one size does not fit all. Do not attempt to do a vegetable-and-fruit-only, or juice fast, without being under the care of a health practitioner.

When meeting with my clients one-on-one or in a group, I am able to offer more extreme detoxes that work quickly and efficiently because I am actually following my clients through the process. Since I don't know you personally, for purposes of this book, the detox here will be a medically sound, generic detox, but will still do the trick of detoxing your body. It will just detox more slowly!

Now, there are seemingly a million detox options out there! Some of them try and convince you that if you just drink a special tea or some crazy concoction every day, or take a supplement, you will be detoxing and transform your body and health. Do not be fooled! Don't follow something you read in a magazine, hear on TV, or see someone on social media doing and experiment on your own as it can be not only a waste of your time and money, but medically very dangerous. (And if you are pregnant, nursing, or undergoing chemo, you should not be detoxing at all.)

I once had a client to whom I gave a medically sound detox and protocol to follow. Because she was a diabetic, her detox was completely different from one I had given her friend. My diabetic client came in the next week with stitches on her head. She followed the detox I gave her friend, rather than following the prescription I gave her, which resulted in her passing out and hitting her head! You always want to follow the advice of your health practitioner or a Certified Health Coach, not a lay person's advice.

Dis-ease begins in the Gut Microbiome

Another reason to detox and eat right is to help improve your gut microbiome. Did you know that you're only as healthy as your gut bacteria?

Our gut bacteria have lots of important jobs and it's paramount to our health and immunity, including but not limited to:

Digesting our food, keeping the integrity of our gut lining, crowding out harmful bacteria, training our immune system to distinguish between friend and foe, helping our set point weight, helps metabolize drugs, produces digestive enzymes, keeps pH balanced, converts sugars to short chain fatty acids for energy, helps absorb nutrients such as iron and calcium, neutralizes cancer causing compounds, synthesizes B complex vitamins, synthesizes fat-soluble vitamins like vitamin K, synthesizes hormones, and according to new studies, is even linked to our mental health.

Scientists are learning more and more about how the microbiome is related to diseases and conditions never linked before. Bacteria also modulate genes and helps determine which diseases get expressed, turning various human genes off and on, which can influence whether or not a disease that you're genetically pre-disposed to actually develops. Modulation of our genes by gut bacteria may explain why inherited diseases don't always afflict family members equally, even in identical twins who have the same genes but different microbes.

Microbial disrupters are everywhere – in the food, the air, the water, the soil, the medication, and products we use. The clinical manifestations of microbial disruptors show up in people of all ages and in a variety of symptoms including but not limited to thyroid problems, asthma, allergies, diabetes, arthritis, eczema and even depression and anxiety. Now a damaged microbiome isn't the only reason people have disease or symptoms related to these conditions, but our gut microbiome does dictate our immunity and combined with genetics, a western diet high in sugar, fat, and processed food, and environmental factors it can create the perfect storm for disease.

The human microbiome is actually the next big frontier in medicine providing answers to why we do get sick, how to heal our bodies and why they are paramount to our overall well-being and health.

Here's what we know:

Things that hurt your Micobiome are:
- Antibiotics
- Pesticides
- Stress
- Medication
- Antibacterial Soaps
- Being too "clean"

Things that HELP your Micobiome are:
- Fermented Foods
- Organic Produce
- Meditation, Sleep
- Probiotics and Prebiotics
- Regular soap and water
- Getting dirty, literally

Probiotics

A daily good probiotic is essential to your microbiome and overall health. Probiotics are live microorganisms or live bacteria which usually come in pill, powder or liquid form.

Probiotics have been used for medicinal purposed for centuries. The Romans used fermented raw milk as an antidote for gastrointestinal infections, and in the 1900's Russian scientist Elie Metchnikoff promoted the use of probiotics after noticing that Bulgarians who consumed lots of fermented products seemed to live longer.

We still don't know all the ways that probiotics can improve health but some of the ways we do know include:

Stimulation of the immune system
Suppression of pathogens
Destruction of toxins
Reduction of inflammation
Reduction of irritable bowel syndrome
Reduction of LDL or "bad" cholesterol

Other conditions that are helped by probiotics include:
Acne
Antibiotic associated diarrhea (AAD)
Irritable Bowel Syndrome (IBS)
Yeast Infections
Urinary Tract Infections (UTI)
Sinus Infections
Leaky gut
Inflammatory bowel disease (IBD)

Conditions that may be helped by probiotics include:
Obesity
Allergies Anxiety/Depression
Autism
Heart Disease
Autoimmune disease
Chronic Fatigue Syndrome

*Note: Be sure to choose a probiotic that has at least 10-50 billion CFU of the two most important groups of probiotic bacteria: Lactobacilli and Bifidobacteria. They should also contain multiple comparible strains of the bacteria designed to work together since different strains have different functions and no one strain can provide all the benefits.

Prebiotics
These are non-digestible foods or ingredients that promote the growth of the beneficial microorganisms in the intestines. In other words they are foods for your gut bacteria like: Oats, bananas, onions, leeks, asparagus, garlic and artichokes.

Synbiotics
These are a combination of probiotics and prebiotics that are found primarily in fermented foods like Kimchi, pickles, Kombucha, Kefir, and sauerkraut. They are good for the gut and also provide a significant amount of live bacteria themselves.

Make sure you are taking all three of these during detox and continue after detox to derive the benefits. Of course it is especially important to include all three for a minimum of three months to a year after taking antibiotics, since it may take up to that long to start working. In general you may need to take probiotics indefinitely to experience continued benefits. Always consult your Nutritionist or Health Care provider.

Before You Detox, Plan Ahead

So you've made the decision to eat right and exercise and improve the quality of your life, the length of your life, God willing, your level of fitness, your health, and your body composition. You've laid your burdens down to God, and asked Him to give you strength and motivation. The next step is a detox.

- First, clean out all the junk and processed food from your kitchen and house. You don't need it around!
- Plan ahead what you are going to eat, how and when you will work out, and when you will spend time with God each day, and do not waver from that! Preparation is key!
- Make the decision to do it. Life is all about decisions.
- Get your measuring tools and do your measurements to monitor your body's progress. Refer to the Fitness chapter to see how to measure.
- Get a water filter and a stainless steel or glass bottle to carry with you.
- Get a journal or use a phone app.
- Purchase quality supplements if you haven't already.
- Buy a wearable tracking device for your exercise.
- Un-junk your body, un-junk your mind, un-junk your life.
- Pray and meditate on God's Word. Ask Him to give you the strength through the Holy Spirit to take care of your temporary earth suit.
- Consider joining my Procoach World Wide Mobile Virtual Coaching Program. (Refer to recommended web sites at the end of the book or go to Robbieraugh.com)
- Consider doing a Social Media detox.

A seven-to-fourteen-day detox is recommended, but quite honestly, what I'm about to have you detox from here is what you should be detoxing from forever. If you choose to go back to some things like dairy and caffeine, be sure you limit them!

By the way, if you don't own a Vitamix blender, you may want to invest in a Ninja blender or NutriBullet for your veggie smoothies and other health drinks because they keep the fiber in and blend it up well!

Guidelines for a 7 to 14-Day Detox

- Eat mostly a plant-based diet. At least 80% plants, no more than 20% fruit.
- Have 3 servings of lean protein a day, plant or animal (make sure the animal products are organic).
- You can have as many plain veggies as you want, preferably raw.
- Have one to three fruits a day (avoid fruit juice).
- Drink lots of filtered water (at least 64 oz.) per day or half of your body weight in ounces of water.
- Cut out processed and junk food (white flour/white sugar, etc.).
- Have only nutrient-dense, whole, gluten-free or sprouted grains, and limit them (depending on your energy output). Remember, not all gluten-free foods are low-glycemic or non-processed.
- Be confident in taking care of your body. Count your blessings. This is the day the Lord has made! Keep your eye on the prize...
- Thank God today for the breath in your lungs... and LIVE the life God gave you to its fullest...with health, energy and vibrancy. And no longer be sick, thick, and tired! You can do this, and anything, through Christ alone.
- If you are a late night snacker, when you feel like eating before bed, DON'T eat, but sleep instead! Avoid late night snacking. In my opinion, this is one of the easiest times to turn away from food and do something different to change your focus. Brushing your teeth is another good remedy because nothing tastes good after you brush your teeth! So, if you're trying to lose weight, don't snack at night. Brush your teeth and go to BED!
- Ditch the alcohol! I find it ironic that one of the things that causes love handles is a six-pack (of beer that is)! But more importantly, the Bible is clear that we should not get drunk.

- Today and every day, ask God to give you strength and self-control to resist the bad foods that cause disease. Focus on all the foods of the earth that God has supplied for us to fuel and feed our bodies—the nutrient-dense foods, the ones you don't need to read a label on!
- Know that the first source of fuel for our body is carbohydrates. The second source of fuel for our body is fat. So when you are trying to lose weight, if you keep eating a lot of carbohydrates, your body is not going to get a chance to use up the fat as fuel. Giving up caffeine isn't forever but you definitely need to do it for detox. After detox you can go back to having caffeine although you probably won't want to. Cut your caffeine intake in half the first three days, gradually decreasing quantity. On day four, cut out caffeine completely. If you go cold turkey on eliminating caffeine (and even sugar) you may get severe headaches, and other adverse symptoms).
- To be part of the journey of health, wellness and fitness, it doesn't matter when you start or if you just started, but when you do start, know you are not alone on this journey as God is with you, and for you.
- Write down your goals and visualize the specific results you want to see (losing 5 pounds etc.).
- Pray.

Stop the vicious cycle of being sick and thick and tired once and for all! Anyone can do anything for 14 days! It will be worth it!

Commit to the Lord whatever you do, and He will establish your plans. (Proverbs 16:3)

What's Wrong with Caffeine?

This is one of the number one questions I get when I am advising people to stay off or cut down on caffeine during detox. Here are the top ten reasons to ditch the caffeine!

1) It can increase your heart rate, elevate blood pressure and can increase the risk for heart problems.
2) Causes blood sugar swings by stimulating a temporary surge in the blood sugar followed by an overproduction of insulin, which then leads to blood sugar plummeting. This all, by the way, leads to weight gain since insulin's message to the body is to store excess sugar as fat!
3) Can cause anxiety, irritability and anxiousness in some people.
4) Stimulates the excretion of stress hormones, which can produce increased levels of anxiety, irritability, muscular tension, and even pain.
5) Causes insomnia which also contributes to weight gain and inability to cope with life stress.
6) Can contribute to female health issues associated with fibrocystic breast disease, exacerbates PMS and menopausal problems, and more.
7) Can contribute to male health issues related to urinary and prostate problems.
8) Causes nutritional deficiencies inhibiting the absorption of some nutrients, can increase urinary excretion of calcium, potassium, magnesium, iron and trace minerals.
9) Can contribute to gastrointestinal problems including but not limited to ulcers, heartburn, and gastroesophageal reflux disease (GERD).
10) Can lead to adrenal exhaustion, which can lead to inflammation and fatigue.

Note: There are of course some health benefits to caffeine, for instance, it increases clarity, concentration and memory. If you feel you have to have it than make sure it's decaf and organic and limit to one cup a day during detox. You can go back on caffeine after detox, but you probably won't want to.

What are the benefits of drinking lemon and warm water?

Incorporate a cup of warm water and a squeeze of half a lemon every morning and reap the following benefits:

- helps balance pH (they are one of the most alkalizing foods for the body)
- antioxidant benefits
- boosts immune system
- aids in digestion
- acts as a natural diuretic
- hydrates body
- aids in weight loss
- helps purify and stimulate gallbladder and liver
- reduces coffee cravings
- freshens breath
- supports immune function
- anti-inflammatory effects
- antimicrobial
- enhances iron absorption in the body
- promotes healing
- supports clear skin

Note: You should continue with this lemon and warm even after detox. Incorporate it in your daily routine for health and wellness.

Sugar Addiction:

Sugar is addictive and increases the amino acid dopamine in our brain for a short time when ingested. This gives us a sensation of pleasure, and of course we end up craving it even more.

Regulation of hormones and neurotransmitters that affect appetite and craving is complex and involves many factors including how quickly food spikes our blood sugars, stress, chemical additives and artificial sweeteners, food allergens and sensitivities, getting enough sleep, nutritional deficiencies which all drive inflammation and more.

To combat sugar addiction we need to detox of course. But also in the long run we need to incorporate these important truths:

1) Stabilize your blood sugar by eating nutrient dense foods including protein and fiber with every meal (raw nuts, seeds, etc). Have smaller meals throughout the day. Eat something every three to

four hours. Avoid eating three hours before bedtime. This will also help your figure!

2) Eliminate sugar and empty carbs that turns into sugar in the body. Avoid all artificial sweeteners as well. Go cold turkey. If you're addicted to alcohol, you don't wean yourself off and have just a little every day, right? That would be a slippery slope! You have to stop completely to stop the cravings and get your brain to reset. Eliminate all refined sugars, sodas, fruit juice, and artificial sweeteners from your diet. These all act like drugs in your body and cause you to crave more. Break the chain!

3) Get seven to eight hours of sleep per night. Research shows that lack of sleep increases cravings.

4) Take your multivitamins and supplements along with eating right, so that your body isn't craving the nutrients, vitamins, and minerals it needs. According to one study, when vitamin D is low, one of the problems (and there are many) is that the hormone that helps turn off your appetite doesn't work as well, and people end up feeling hungry all the time. Also know that omega-3s have many benefits, including helping with brain function, insulin control and reducing inflammation.

Do you not know that your body is a temple of the Holy Spirit, who is in you, whom you have received from God? You are not your own; you were bought at a price. Therefore honor God with your body. (1 Corinthians 6:19-20)

Forget what is behind and straining toward what is ahead. Press on toward the goal to win the prize which God has called me heavenward in Christ Jesus. (Philippians 3:13-14 [paraphrased])

Maintain self-control:
Self-control comes from giving God control. It's not honorable to be mastered by anything other than the Master! You will always lose when you lose self-control. We need self-control in all arenas of our life.

Here's the truth: you may have cravings or just want to indulge once in a while. But stop and think, is it worth feeling and looking awful for temporary pleasure? We can say, "I love doughnuts," but that doesn't mean they are good for us or that we need to eat them! I'm pretty sure Mick Jagger wasn't talking about this subject when he sang, "You can't always get what you want" but it applies; we can't and shouldn't always get what we want.

If it's white, don't bite! If there is sugar, gluten, or dairy, it won't make you merry! Get the picture? You should get to the point where you just wake up and don't want to feel bad anymore.

Remember: You don't even know how bad you feel until you start feeling good physically, mentally, and emotionally!

> *And God is faithful; He will not let you be tempted beyond what you can bear. But when you are tempted, He will provide a way out so that you can stand up under it. (1 Corinthians 10:12)*

And remember if you go outside the lines, remember, a bend in the road is not the end of the road when GOD is involved. He is sovereign!

The Raw Truth Recharge 7 to 14-Day Detox

You will eat: The nutrient dense foods of the earth that God created.

You will give up: All CATS (caffeine, alcohol, tobacco, and sugar) and chemicals, preservatives, carcinogens, and everything else that's bad for you or that you need to read a label on. (See list below).

Also avoid all processed food, pesticides, preservatives, dairy (organic eggs ok), artificial sweeteners, soda, fruit juice, baked goods, junk food, red meat/animal products, and white potatoes.

What to Eat During Your Detox, Week One:

Include Protein: Have three protein (organic animal or plant) servings per day with veggies. Remember plant-based protein is preferred.

Plant protein options: ¼ to ½ cup beans, legumes, lentils, hummus (with no sugar), Non-GMO Tofu, Tempeh, and greens like kale/spinach etc.

For a protein substitute, use a plant-based protein powder like Sun Warrior or Vega, using a half cup or one whole cup of unsweetened almond milk per serving. Vegetarians only can have five to ten raw organic walnuts or almonds per day.

Animal protein options: Organic eggs, organic chicken, fish, or turkey. Avoid red meat during detox. A serving size is 4-8 ounces of meat per meal (or two to three eggs). You can use the palm of your hand to measure the serving sizes.

Eat and drink only organic plant products and animal products (make certain they do not contain pesticides, steroids, antibiotics, or carcinogens).

Fish and Seafood: Make sure you stick to the deep-sea fish like wild salmon, tuna, swordfish and shark. Limit to a couple of times a month if you are concerned about mercury.

Include Grains:
You can have one slice of Ezekiel Sprouted Grain Bread or a quarter-cup of Ezekiel Sprouted Grain Cereal two to three times per week (on workout days).

You can also substitute for a low glycemic gluten free bread.

No pastas, rice, crackers, potatoes, quinoa, etc., and no other bread). If you are trying to lose weight it's good to give up grains for 6 weeks under the care of a health professional only.

Include Healthy Fats: Use sparingly one to two servings of *one* of the following per day-

- Cold-pressed olive, macadamia, walnut, sunflower, grape seed or coconut oil. Use a spray bottle or use sparingly.
- ½ of a small avocado.
- One cup of unsweetened almond milk, flax milk, or coconut milk. Unsweetened chocolate or vanilla are okay as well.
- One teaspoon to one tablespoon of chia, flax, pumpkin, or sunflower seeds.
- Include five to twelve raw nuts, preferably almonds or walnuts.

Include Veggies:
Eat as many plain organic veggies as you want all day long. Raw vegetables are preferable, but cooked, roasted, grilled, or steamed are okay as well. Just do not overcook them.

Green smoothies are okay unless you take anti-coagulants.

Include Fruits:
Limit to one or two servings of organic fruit per day which are high in antioxidants, for example, blackberries, blueberries, raspberries, elderberries, strawberries.

Drinks:
Drink at least half your body weight in ounces of filtered water per day. You can flavor your water with cucumbers, ginger, lemon, etc.

Have one cup of warm water with a half-squeeze of fresh lemon every morning.

One Immune-Boosting Green Smoothie a day. I suggest using a Vitamix and use Organic Spinach or Kale, water base, one fruit and any vegetables you want. You can also add chia seeds, lemon or spices. If you don't want a smoothie you can have your greens in a raw salad, just get them in everyday! I love Powershot Raw Organic Powder Greens.

Herbal decaf green tea or other herbal decaf teas are okay as well.

What to Eat During Your Detox, Week Two:
Same as Week One, but now you eliminate dairy, potatoes, grains, flours, bread (none, not even Ezekiel), nuts, seeds, nut butters, and beans.

Continue to have 3 servings of organic protein a day. Avoid red meat.

Optional: plant protein powder (plant protein only), one to two servings per day unless otherwise instructed. Use Sun Warrior or Vega brand with filtered water only. No almond or coconut milk.

Drink warm water with a squeeze of half a lemon every day. This will cleanse your palate and also to cleanse the gall bladder, helping to metabolize fat.

Exercise: Light to moderate intensity is okay, depending on how you feel. No vigorous exercise.

Considerations

Not taking in enough nutrients can result in low blood-sugar levels, dehydration, fatigue, dizziness and nausea. Remember: pregnant or nursing women should not detox. Neither should young children.

Sample Menu:

Breakfast: Pea Protein and Powershot smoothie with 1 TBS of chia seeds and your favorite unsweetened Nut or Coconut Milk.

Lunch: Arugula Salad with low mercury Tuna, Wild Salmon or Chick Peas or lentils

Midday snack: 9-12 nuts or ¼ cup of hummus and veggies.

Dinner: A Vegetarian Dish (see Lentil Walnut Salad in recipes), or Broccoli with Wild Salmon, and a Cabbage Salad.

*Then fast for 12-16 hours. If your last meal was 7pm then don't eat until 7am the next morning!

Raw Truth Tips :

- The first three to four days will be rough if you are used to drinking a lot of coffee and eating sugar. Once you detox from that, and break the chain, it will be easy. By day five you will feel better, and your energy will increase dramatically! Remember, nothing that's good in life is easy.
- You will be a little tired. Keep busy, but rest when you can.
- You can add hot sauce or any spices you want during detox.
- Use our Detox Soup and Detox Salad Dressing recipes to make soup and salad.
- You should never be hungry if you are eating enough vegetables! The more you eat, the higher your metabolism, and the more fat you burn, so don't go hungry!
- Drink all the water recommended per day. It will help you lose more weight and flush out toxins.

- Prepare your veggies, soup, etc. in advance!! Preparation is key!
- Use the Internet to search vegan recipes and then eliminate oils, sauces, etc.
- Stay connected to others who are doing this with you, but don't share this with others, as anyone detoxing should be under the care of a health professional/coach.
- Eat food, not food-like things.
- If you are trying to eliminate fat on your body it makes perfect sense for you to cut down on the amount of fat you put into your body.

What kinds of symptoms can I expect to have during detox?

As I mentioned, it is normal to experience some temporary adverse side effects from the body getting rid of the toxins and chemicals. These symptoms can include:

- Headaches
- Lethargy
- Temporary aches and pains
- Nausea or vomiting
- Slight weakness (so don't exercise vigorously)
- Irritability
- Flu-like symptoms
- Constipation

Just remember, if you experience headaches and these kind of symptoms from giving up sugar and junk food, imagine what they're doing to your body every day?

Soon you will start feeling amazing, around day five. And you won't know how bad you feel on a regular basis until you start feeling good!

Relief from detox symptoms

Your body needs to go through the detox process to feel better on the other side. Allow the symptoms to happen. Don't mask the symptoms with pain medication. If you need to slow down the process of the detox, incorporate more protein, healthy fats and easily digestible healthy foods like avocados, coconut oil, raw nuts, sunflower seeds, etc. Also remember to lay your burdens down to the King! He will give you the strength you need to persevere! Do not be tempted to go back to processed foods, sugar and caffeine. Break the chain! Pray.

What to Eat Post-Detox, Weeks Three through Eight

Continue to stay off the junk, processed food, chemicals, carcinogens, etc. Do everything as before, but you can now add the following back in:

Dairy: Eat in moderation and only orgranic.

Caffeine: If you are adding back caffeine, start with decaf first. Better yet, try yerba mate tea.

Low-GI food, one serving per day: A quarter- to a half-cup of beans/legumes (red, garbanzo, lima, mung, pinto, black, baked [no sugar], edamame, lentils, red kidney, or soybeans) or a half or one small sweet potato/yam, winter squash, spaghetti, acorn, or pumpkin squash.

Grains, either sprouted or low-glycemic gluten-free: One to two times per week. Avoid for 6 weeks if trying to lose weight.

Healthy Fats: Use sparingly one to two servings of <u>one</u> of the following per day-

- One to two teaspoons of cold-pressed olive, macadamia, walnut, sunflower, grape seed or coconut oil. Use a spray bottle or use sparingly.
- ¼ to ½ of a small avocado.
- One cup of unsweetened almond milk, flax milk, or coconut milk. Even unsweetened chocolate or vanilla is okay.
- One teaspoon to one tablespoon of chia, flax, pumpkin, or sunflower seeds.
- Include five to twelve raw nuts, preferably almonds or walnuts.

"Unhealthy" Fats – Milk/Cheese/Yogurt: – if you must consume, limit to a couple times per week or less and make sure it's organic..

Avoid cheese and milk products as much as possible, but if you have to have it, limit to a couple times per week or less, and make sure it's low- or non-fat and preferably organic.

Fish and Seafood: Make sure you stick to the deep-sea fish like wild salmon, tuna, swordfish and shark.

Note: Keep the water and lemon going, start taking supplements, and get plenty of rest. Exercise five to seven days per week (weights, cardio and flexibility). And don't forget the water!

Exercise 5-7 days per week (more frequent, and longer is better):
Cardio: 30-60 minutes of moderate to intense cardio 4 to 5 days per week.

Weight Lifting: 3 days per week, 60 minutes, all muscle groups, 8-12 reps to the point of failure. Optional: Divide muscle groups 4-5 alternating days.

Mind/Body/Flexibility (like Yoga): 2 to 3 days per week.

Don't forget breakfast!
The old adage is true: Breakfast really is the most important meal of the day. You will feel amazing all day long with the perfect amount of carbs, proteins and fresh foods to start your day. Get up just a few minutes earlier and try some of these ideas that don't take a lot of time.

Remember God wants us to take care of our temple and feed it good foods of the earth that HE created! And you don't need to read a label when you are eating food of the earth like an apple!

A breakfast protein drink is probably easiest when you have a time crunch. I use unsweetened Vanilla Almond Milk Plant Powder or Pea Protein Powder. I also love organic spinach, apple or clementine, lemon, cinnamon, and water shakes! You can even throw in some chia or ground flax seeds for extra fiber, omega-3s, protein, etc. (I prefer chia over flax). Try 1 tsp. of Powershot Organic Raw Green Powder to get a dozens greens in one shot.

Steel-Cut Oats are another great breakfast option, which take a little more work, but is everything you need to feel great all morning long. Have a bowl of steel-cut oats, with a handful of almonds, blueberries, or raspberries. You can make the steel-cut oats the night before to save some time in the morning. You can really kick this breakfast option into high gear by adding a cup of delicious green tea to get your metabolism really kicking by mid-morning. This is the perfect combination of protein, carbs and antioxidants to get your body up and running right away.

The Egg Bake (frittata) listed in the recipe section is another great breakfast, which can be made ahead of time and refrigerated to keep all week long. Of course veggie omelets are always a healthy option too.

Sautéed Spinach in vinegar is another great choice packed with vitamins and minerals for a power breakfast. Or you can make a spinach shake!

Snacks of protein and fiber are helpful once or twice a day in between meals. My emergency "go to's" are a protein shake, or about 9-12 nuts, or some vegetables, or hummus and veggies. The point is to keep your blood sugar stabilized.

Supplements and Medications:
Continue taking your medications/supplements as directed by your physician or another health practitioner.

Before workout:
Try drinking this Energizer Smoothie:

> 1-2 cups of Kale, Spinach (or 1 tsp. of poweshot)
> 1 stalk of celery, ½ lemon,
> a dash of cinnamon, water, 2 carrots,
> ¼ cup of berries, ice –
> Truly this is better than caffeine!! You will be flying!

After workout:
Give yourself a healthy snack, like raw veggies and a quarter-cup of hummus, or a protein smoothie with chocolate plant protein powered,

unsweetened vanilla, nut or coconut milk, ¼ cup of berries, ice, and filtered water.

*Note an extra protein snack is okay if you are trying to gain muscle mass. Otherwise to build muscle and lifting weights, omit the fourth serving of protein. Be sure to take your supplements and drink ½ of your body weight in ounces of water per day!

Write down everything you drink and eat and how you feel!
Meditate on:

> *Whoever wants to be my disciple must deny themselves and take up their cross daily and follow me. (Luke 9:23)*

> *Be diligent in these matters; give yourself wholly to them, so that everyone may see your progress. (1 Timothy 4:15)*

In summary
Detox seasonally but especially if you have any of the following symptoms:

- Lack of energy
- Trouble losing weight or keeping it off
- Acne or other skin ailments
- Achy joints and inflammation
- Need caffeine to get up in the morning
- Need medication to go to sleep at night
- Have digestive issues
- Sugar cravings
- You feel bloated
- You feel spiritually starved

Avoid Inflammatory Foods:

- Dairy
- Sugar and sugar-containing foods or food-like things.
- Trans fats

- Red meat and processed meat
- Alcohol
- Refined grains
- Artificial food additives
- Allergens (any food you are allergic to or have a sensitivity to)
- Animal products that were injected with antibiotics and hormones
- Cooking oils (corn, cottonseed, safflower, soy, sunflower)
- Artificial food additives
- Food-like things

Incorporate Anti-Inflammatory Foods:
- Wild Alaskan salmon
- Kelp, kale, spinach
- Blueberries, strawberries, blackberries
- Green tea
- Turmeric
- Sweet potato
- Garlic
- EVOO (Extra Virgin Olive Oil) – cold pressed is best
- Ginger
- Watercress
- Cruciferous vegetables

Juicing and Blending:
As I mentioned, I prefer the Vitamix, but the Ninja or NutriBullet will also suffice. You need to keep the fiber in the juice so don't take it out.

Note: If you are used to taking in a lot of toxins and you are sick, the toxins may release quickly from your body, making your detox symptoms even stronger. Green smoothies or drinks without protein added are a wonderful detoxifier, but you need to be careful if you are on certain medications like anticoagulants since the vitamin K can interfere with the medication.

One of my favorite green drinks is called PowerShot! It's a Raw Organic power of a dozen greens including wheat grass which you can mix just 1tsp. in your water or favorite nut milk and get all of the phytonutrients you need for the day. It's delicious even by itself! I even mix in with my pea protein powder. See the link for this at the back of the book.

The Mind is a Battlefield – Detox Spiritually

Take the time to cleanse or detox your mind and spirit. Remember that the enemy will try and make you fail! Cleanse your mind and detox all of the negative self-sabotaging thoughts running like a tape recorder in your head and remember how God wants you to take care of your "mobile home." Remind yourself that we need energy and vibrant health to go out and do His will for our lives.

Meditating on God's Word will actually affect your body. It will reduce your stress and improve your health.

Remember self-control is a Fruit of the Spirit. You need to practice it and you have the power of the Holy Spirit inside of you to do it. Self-control is also like exercise, the easier you do it, the easier it becomes and the stronger you get.

> *Finally, brothers and sisters, whatever is true, whatever is noble, whatever is right, whatever is pure, whatever is lovely, whatever is admirable—if anything is excellent or praiseworthy—think about such things. (Philippians 4:8)*

There is hope in God's truth. Keep pressing toward the goal.

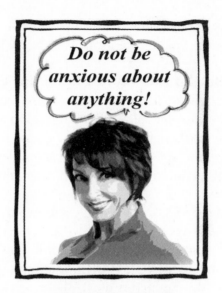

TRUTH SIX

Manage Stress
4:6 It!

Be anxious for nothing, but in everything by prayer and supplication with thanksgiving, let your requests be made known to God; and the peace of God, which surpasses all understanding, will guard your hearts and minds through Christ Jesus. (Phil 4:6-7)

S TRESS—WE ALL HAVE it! And you need to manage it, because it will affect your health adversely if you don't, no matter how well you eat or exercise! Truly, the best way to manage and reduce stress is to just lay your burdens down at God's feet because God is the God of miracles. A bend in the road is not the end of the road when you know God! "Let go, let God" is a cliché, but it's so very true. I tell my patients to "4-6 it": *Philippians 4-6* tells us, *Do not be anxious about anything, but in every situation, by prayer and petition, with thanksgiving, present your requests to God.*

You know, as a nurse, I used to work in the emergency room. Talk about stress! Do you think I had stress? Absolutely. After working in the ER, oftentimes when people around me would get stressed out, I would say, "Well, no one died..." meaning it's not that bad. And when you give it all to God, and you trust in His sovereignty, you know there isn't much you can control, or need to control.

There will be times in your life when you may feel alone and in the dark, and there will be demonic activity around us. But Jesus can cause the enemy to flee when you completely submit to Him. The key is we have to submit to Him and keep our eyes on Him alone. Pray without ceasing. God knows your needs, He knows your problems, He knows your pain, He sees your sorrows. He's God! Did you ever try and pray but you were so stressed out you couldn't even formulate your thoughts to pray? Like you didn't even know how to pray, it was so big? You don't have to have the words, you know. God knows... He's God.

There are four risk factors to disease. They are:

1) Stress
2) Lack of sleep
3) Obesity
4) Eating sub-optimal food (processed food, junk food, sugar, etc.)

Did you notice what the number one risk factor is? That's right—stress! Stress affects your whole body and your mind.

Stress and Weight
Long-term stress can make you fat, studies have found. When you're chronically stressed, your body is flooded with stress hormones, which stimulate fat cells deep in the abdomen to increase in size and encourage fat storage. And stress hormones spark your appetite, making you likely to overeat.

> Consider it pure joy, my brothers, whenever you face trials of
> many kinds, because you know that the testing of your faith

develops perseverance. Perseverance must finish its work so that you may be mature and complete, not lacking anything. (James 1:2-4)

At times of stress in our lives, our body produces a hormone called cortisol. Cortisol increases blood pressure and blood sugar, and lowers your immune system. If you remain in a stressful state for a prolonged period of time, you can experience weight gain, and your health can be negatively affected (allowing disease to creep in). When cortisol is released, your metabolism is slowed down and your blood sugars are elevated. It then stimulates deep abdominal fat to accept and store fat, and to make matters worse, you start craving chocolate, caffeine, high-glycemic and high-fat foods. Stress affects all of us. It fools with our emotions, prevents us from thinking logically, and robs us of energy.

Humble yourselves, therefore, under God's mighty hand, that He may lift you up in due time. Cast all your anxiety on Him because He cares for you. Be self-controlled and alert. Your enemy the devil prowls around like a roaring lion looking for someone to devour. Resist him, standing firm in the faith, because you know that your brothers throughout the world are undergoing the same kind of sufferings. (1 Peter 5:6-9)

The Fight-or-Flight Response

Stress can trigger the body's response to perceived threat or danger, which is called the fight-or-flight response. During this reaction, certain hormones like adrenaline and cortisol are released, speeding the heart rate, slowing digestion, shunting blood flow to major muscle groups, and changing various other autonomic nervous functions, giving the body a burst of energy and strength. Originally named for its ability to enable us to physically fight or run away when faced with danger, it's now activated in situations where neither response is appropriate, like in traffic or during a stressful day at work. Chronic stress can lead to health problems and of course disease.

Do Not Worry

Remember, in Matthew 6:25, God tells us not to worry about those things that God promises to supply. Worry can affect your health negatively, cause the object of worry to consume your thoughts, disrupt your productivity, negatively affect the way you treat others, and negatively affect your ability to trust God. It's okay to be concerned but worry can paralyze you, and concern can inspire you to take action.

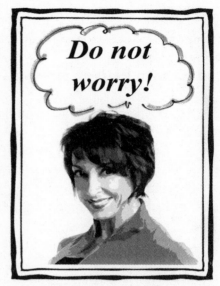

Remember, if God leads you to it, He will lead you through it! I have always remembered this when I'm going on the air or doing anything outside my comfort zone. I have to remind myself that He placed me there!

Stress and Health

When faced with chronic stress and an over activated autonomic nervous system, people begin to experience physical symptoms. The first symptoms are relatively mild, like chronic headaches and increased susceptibility to colds. With more exposure to chronic stress, however, more serious health problems may develop. These stress-influenced conditions include, but are not limited to:

- depression
- diabetes
- hair loss
- heart disease
- hyperthyroidism
- obesity
- obsessive-compulsive or anxiety disorder
- sexual dysfunction
- tooth and gum disease
- ulcers
- some cancers

In fact, it's been estimated that as many as 90% of doctor's visits are for symptoms that are at least partially stress-related!

7 Truths to Relieve Stress

1. Pray, and read God's Word. "4-6" it!
2. Get enough sleep.
3. Go for a walk or work out.
4. Take natural supplements like St. John's Wort.
5. Shut down electronically.
6. Cut yourself some slack or develop an "oh well" attitude on the small stuff.
7. Spend time with a good friend.

And remember, a bend in the road is not the end of the road! There is always something to find hope and joy in.

7 Truths To Help You Turn Things Around

1) Pray. God is the God of the impossible. He can make things happen supernaturally. It doesn't matter how many times you've failed, or what statistics say, God is with you and He can lift you up. Lean on God. If you want to get lean, lean on the Lord.

   For I know the plans I have for you, declares the Lord, plans to prosper you and not harm you, plans to give you hope and a future. (Jeremiah 29:11)

2) Lean on your family and friends. When the Beatles wrote, "I get by with a little help from my friends," they knew what they were talking about. Those relationships are important.
3) Have your blood checked. You may be deficient in vitamins, which can affect your mood and your ability to handle stress.
4) Take supplements that contain ginseng, rose hips, and St. John's Wort, but be careful if you're taking medication. Check the contraindications.
5) Exercise!! Boost your mood!

6) Put things in perspective. Don't sweat the small stuff, and as they say, it's all small stuff. If your heart is beating, you have breath in your lungs, and a meal for the day, you're doing great!
7) Realize the sovereignty of God. Consider the fact that some things are just out of your control, but that He is in control. It doesn't help to worry about them or let them get you down. Let go, let God, lay your burdens down and pray.

*If you don't feel better seek professional help. Call your doctor or a counselor or therapist.

Do not let your hearts be troubled. Trust in God, Trust also in Me. (John 14:1)

Thankfulness!

When praying, don't forget to count your blessings and thank God for them first and foremost! I am thankful for little things every day, like the breath in my lungs and the beat of my heart. I am thankful for my family, our beautiful girls who are gifts from God, and my friends who are like family. I am thankful for our health, food, heat, a roof over our heads, clothes on our backs, and more than we need. I am thankful for my friends who I don't know that well who have touched me in some way. I'm thankful for all the blessings and ministries God has given me. I'm thankful that I get to wake up every day, do what I love, and feel that it matters. I'm thankful for all the time I have been able to spend with loved ones. I am thankful that I was able to help my mom, sister and dad during their life and escort them out of this world, with God's love and tenderness. I'm thankful that my Mom taught me how to love through her own sacrifices and beautiful demonstration of love. I am thankful that Mom instilled in me that with God all things are possible. I am most thankful that Jesus died... so I could live. Realize the sovereignty of God. Consider the fact that some things are just out of your control and it doesn't help to worry about them or let them get you down.

In summary:

Allow God to give you peace and rest. Cast your cares on the One who cares. Worship instead of worry! You don't have to fight your own battles. God's grace and power can make things happen with ease that you can't bring about no matter how hard you try. It's so freeing to say, "I don't have a clue what's going to happen but God does, so I'm not going to worry about it."

Jim Rohn said, "The walls we build around us to keep sadness out also keep out the joy."

John Lennon said, "Everything will be OK in the end, if it's not OK, it's the end."

C.S. Lewis said, "There are far, far better things ahead than we leave behind."

Francis Chan said, "Worry implies we don't quite trust that God is big enough, powerful enough or loving enough to take care of what's happening in our lives.

Stress says the things we are involved in are important enough to merit our impatience, our lack of grace toward others or our tight grip of control."

It all comes down to this, it doesn't matter where we are in our life right now when we know God, because we can be content that it's exactly where we are supposed to be. When we seek God with all of our soul, all of our strength and all of our might, He will make our paths straight. What's there to worry about with that?

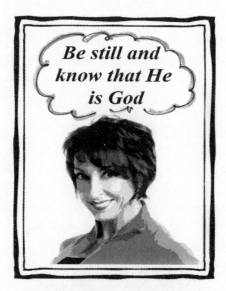

TRUTH SEVEN

Sleep
Be Still

Come to Me, all who are weary and heavy-laden, and I will give you rest. (Matthew 11:28)

I AM ONE OF those people who just doesn't function well at 6 a.m., although I'm up at that time just about every morning. I never want to go to bed at night because I feel great at night and I'm most productive at night. Like right now, I'm writing this book, and it's almost midnight! When I had my two beautiful babies, it was me who got up several times a night to feed and change them. My husband Jeff was snoring away in a deep sleep. Seriously, a tornado could come through the house and he wouldn't wake up! I on the other hand am the opposite. I would wake up when my girls were babies if I heard a little peep from them while they slept, and I'm still like that today.

So I have to be very deliberate and do the math to make sure I get to bed on time, so I can get enough sleep, because if I don't I can't operate on all cylinders the next day. Lack of sleep affects everything we do negatively. Sleep deprivation affects our mood, our memory, our ability to concentrate or process things, our ability to handle stress, causes adrenal fatigue, health problems, decision making, and of course as I've mentioned, it can affect our weight!

Too Little Sleep Affects Appetite

A study that recorded the sleep patterns of 9,000 people indicated that those who averaged only six hours of sleep per night were 27% more likely to be overweight than those who slept seven to nine hours. Study participants who averaged five hours of sleep per night were 73% more likely to be overweight.

How does a lack of sleep contribute to feelings of hunger? Scientists say that a lack of sleep leads to hormonal disturbances, causing the hormones leptin and ghrelin to get out of balance. When you are sleep-deprived, your body produces too little leptin, the hormone that tells you you're full, and too much ghrelin, the hormone that tells you you're hungry.

The next day, those hormones cause you to crave bad carbs and sugars, eat more, and burn fewer calories while making you less able to feel full. With all these hormones stacked against you, no wonder you are having a hard time fighting temptation of your guilty pleasures!

Skimping on sleep can derail your metabolism as well. In a study at the University of Chicago, people who got four hours of sleep or less a night had more difficulty processing carbohydrates. When you're exhausted, your body lacks the energy to perform its normal, day-to-day functions, which include burning calories, so your metabolism is automatically lowered.

In simple terms: You can eat healthy and exercise all you want, but if your sleep isn't dialed in, you are wasting your time.

We need to consciously shut off the electronics at night to get sleep! Even a small light on in the room from the clock can disrupt our sleep according to researchers.

God's Word commands us to rest and to be still. In fact, in the Bible, there are several references to Jesus resting.

One of my favorite verses is Psalm 46:10, *"Be still and know that I am God."*. God reminds me to stop and hear His voice.

A song by MercyMe, "Word of God Speak," speaks right to me. In that song, the lyrics say:

I'm finding myself at a loss for words
And the funny thing is it's okay
The last thing I need is to be heard
But to hear what You would say

I love that verse and this song because sometimes we just need to slow down and take the time to think and pray and let God speak to us, in silence. Plateaus can be spiritual as well as physical. We hit a plateau spiritually when we just aren't growing in our faith. Sometimes God gently nudges us to be still and hear Him; other times He uses other measures to get our attention. But all of the time we need to be still and dive into His Word. My quiet time with Him is in the early morning and late at night when everyone else is sleeping. But I'm also talking to Him and praying all day long!

New Sleep Recommendations
In February 2015, The National Sleep Foundation convened experts from the fields of sleep, anatomy, and physiology, as well as pediatrics, neurology, gerontology and gynecology, to reach a consensus from the broadest range of scientific disciplines. The panel revised the recommended sleep ranges for all age groups. A summary of the new recommendations includes:

- Newborns (0 to 3 months): Sleep range narrowed to 14 to 17 hours each day (previously it was 12 to 18)
- Infants (4 to 11 months): Sleep range widened two hours to 12 to 15 hours (previously it was 14 to 15)
- Toddlers (1 to 2 years): Sleep range widened by one hour to 11 to 14 hours (previously it was 12 to 14)
- Preschoolers (3 to 5): Sleep range widened by one hour to 10 to 13 hours (previously it was 11 to 13)
- School age children (6 to 13): Sleep range widened by one hour to 9 to 11 hours (previously it was 10 to 11)
- Teenagers (14 to 17): Sleep range widened by one hour to 8 to 10 hours (previously it was 8.5 to 9.5)

- Younger adults (18 to 25): Sleep range is 7 to 9 hours (new age category)
- Adults (26 to 64): Sleep range did not change and remains 7 to 9 hours
- Older adults (65+): Sleep range is 7 to 8 hours (new age category)

7 Raw Truths to Help You Get a Good Night's Sleep

1) Take a warm bath, hot tub, or sauna.
2) Take natural supplements like melatonin and St. John's Wort.
3) Pray.
4) Write down things you need to remember for tomorrow and keep it by your bedside so that you aren't waking up worrying you will forget them.
5) Exercise.
6) Turn off all electronics and light in the room.
7) Read God's Word.

And we know that in all things God works for the good of those who love Him, who have been called according to His purpose. (Romans 8:28)

SUMMARY OF RAW TIPS AND TRUTHS

H ERE ARE SOME **Raw Tips and Truths** to remember about staying healthy and fit:

1. PRAY. God is faithful and God's Word tells us we should *ask, seek, knock*. Remember, God wants us to take care of our earthly bodies, so that we can go out and do His work!
2. Make sure you are eating right and drinking enough water, because if you are not, this will negatively affect your energy level. Avoid all processed food, sugar, white flour, trans fats, hydrogenated oils, soda pop, etc. Focus on the foods of the earth that God created! Eat mostly an organic plant-based diet. Avoid GMO foods.
3. Get adequate rest so you have energy not just to make it through the day but also to make a difference in the lives of the people around you!
4. Work out consistently and at least 5 to 7 days per week. People who work out only one day a week (called weekend warriors), have a tendency to get injured. Don't be one of them!
5. If at all possible, try and get a workout buddy so that you can push each other and hold each other accountable when one wants to slack off.
6. Just show up and start! Lace up your running shoes and hit the streets; get to the gym; do whatever you can to make it happen. I love the gym because it's like the "no excuse zone." You know once you get there you're not going to stand around doing nothing in the midst of everyone else working hard. If you can't get to the gym, grab a friend and get outside!
7. Focus on the results—you obtain results every time you work out. If you have to remind yourself every 15 minutes during your workout why you are there, so be it! Whatever works! In any event, don't let excuses get in your way. You need to work out as if your life depends on it, because in so many ways it does. It's not by accident that Philippians 4:13 is my favorite verse! You can do this!

8. If you think you don't have the time or money to eat right and exercise, remember you will spend the time and the money either way. You will either spend the time and the money preventing disease, or you will you spend the time and the money treating disease. Which is better for you?

9. Remember if you want to get lean, lean on the Lord! And have self-control!

10. Have an attitude of gratitude, and don't sweat the small stuff. Let go, let God.

Some Final Thoughts

- God loves us no matter what the scale says, but He wants us to be healthy, vibrant and full of energy, so that we can go out and do His will for our lives.

- Are you healthy? Just because you are absent from disease does not mean you are well.

- High blood pressure, high cholesterol, strokes, type 2 diabetes, most cancers, and heart attacks are preventable. Most people do not have any signs and symptoms before they have a heart attack.

- Your genes are not your fate! Break the chain!

- You are supposed to consume food; food is not supposed to consume you!

- You crave what you eat! So make the right choices!

- It's not honorable to be ruled by anything other than God.

- Take charge of your future. If you don't, someone else surely will, at a price.

- No one has time to exercise; you simply make time because it's that important.

- Whatever it is that you give up to make time to exercise, you can do much better afterwards.

- When you are too tired to work out, remember that energy produces energy!! Many times you are tired because you have not exercised!

- Remember there are no sweatless quickies!

- What you weigh right now means far less to me as a health professional than what you're doing for your health on a daily basis.

- God cares more about the condition of our heart than the condition of our body, however we need to take care of the body He gave us! Our "mobile home."
- Nothing changes if nothing changes and yesterday you said tomorrow! Just start!

Do not be wise in your own eyes; fear the Lord and shun evil. This will bring health to your body and nourishment to your bones. (Proverbs 3:7-8)

THE RAW TRUTH RECHARGE RECIPES

Recipe Contributions:

Valerie Bielmeier
Keri Cardinale
Michelle Fisher
Lara Frendjian
Donna Fournier

Jeff Raugh
Robbie Raugh
Beth Skorka Zola
Ann Marie Landel

Main Dishes

Coconut Chicken with Pineapple Salsa

Ingredients
2 organic chicken breasts, cut in half lengthwise and pounded thin
½ cup organic coconut oil, melted
1 cup organic unsweetened shredded coconut flakes
Sea salt and ground black pepper
4 Tbsp. coconut oil

Salsa:
1 can pineapple chunks, drained
2 Tbsp. chopped cilantro leaves
1 Tbsp. diced red onion
2 tsp. organic coconut palm sugar
1 Tbsp. minced jalapeno pepper
3 Tbsp. diced red bell pepper

Directions

1. Sprinkle both sides of the chicken breasts with sea salt and ground black pepper.
2. Put approximately 2 tablespoons of melted coconut oil in a pie plate. Put coconut flakes in another bowl.
3. Dip each breast in the oil until coated on both sides, then put in the coconut bowl and press down to make the coconut stick. Turn to coat on both sides.
4. Heat the other 2 tablespoons of coconut oil in a nonstick pan on medium-high heat. Cook chicken in oil for approximately 3-5 minutes on each side.
5. Place all salsa ingredients in a bowl and mix well.
6. Top each piece of chicken with the salsa mixture.

Raw Energy Cereal

Organic Ingredients

1 Tbsp. chia seeds
1 Tbsp. of hulled hemp seeds
1 Tbsp. of ground flax seeds
1 Tbsp. of sunflower seeds
1 Tbsp. of sprouted pumpkin seed
1 Tbsp. of white mulberries
½ cup of fresh raspberries
3 drops of stevia
2 Tbsp. of unsweetened coconut flakes
¼ cup of slivered almonds
1 cup of unsweetened almond milk

Directions

1. Mix the first 4 ingredients in a bowl with one cup almond milk, then let sit while you mix the remainder of the ingredients.
2. Add the remainder all at once ten minutes later.

Cupcake Egg Bake

Ingredients
½ carton of egg whites or 1 dozen organic eggs and/or egg whites
½ cup chopped spinach
1 medium onion chopped
1 medium green pepper chopped
A dash of non-GMO soy bacon bits (optional)
1 cup of salsa
Salt and pepper to taste

Directions
1. Preheat oven to 350 degrees.
2. Spray each cupcake container with EVOO.
3. Fill each cup with egg.
4. Add 1 teaspoon or more of salsa.
5. Add spinach, onions and peppers, and a couple shakes of soy bacon bits in each cupcake.
6. Salt and pepper to taste.
7. Bake at 350 degrees for 20 to 25 minutes.
8. Top with salsa after cooled.
9. Freeze and use as needed.

Eggplant Parmesan in Coconut Oil and Coconut Flakes

Ingredients
2 large eggplants (trim tops and bottoms)
1 Tbsp. olive oil
1 bag of organic unsweetened small coconut flakes
4 organic eggs, beaten

Directions
1. Cut eggplant length-wise into thin slices.
2. Dip into beaten egg and then dip in coconut flakes.
3. Saute in pan until golden brown.
Note: you can also make with recipe using your favorite fish.

Tofu Bake

Organic Ingredients
2 blocks tofu, sliced
¼ cup Bragg's Liquid Aminos
1 Tbsp. olive oil
Juice of 2 limes
1-inch piece of ginger, grated
Fresh ground pepper

Directions
1. Preheat oven to 375 degrees.
2. In baking dish, mix oil, Bragg's, lime juice, ginger, and pepper.
3. Lay tofu slices into mixture, covering both sides.
4. Line up tofu in dish.
5. Bake at 375 degrees for half an hour.

Peanut Sesame Noodles

Organic Ingredients
1 lb Sprouted Grain or gluten-free pasta, or kelp noodles
3 Tbsp. Tahini
1 Tbsp. of peanut or almond butter
1 tsp. of coconut nectar
2 Tbsp. of rice vinegar
2 Tbsp. of soy sauce
1 tsp. of sesame and/or crushed nuts

Directions
1. Prepare pasta as instructed on package.
2. Whisk together all other ingredients and serve over warm pasta.

Robbie's Frittata (Egg Bake)

Ingredients
¼ cup of chopped onions
¼ cup of chopped green and red peppers
¼ cup of chopped spinach
¼ cup of chopped mushrooms
1 dozen organic eggs and ½ carton of egg whites

Directions
1. Preheat oven to 350 degrees.
2. Coat pan with coconut oil or EVOO.
3. Mix eggs or egg whites together.
4. Put egg mixture in the bottom of the 9x5 inch pan or cupcake pan.
5. Bake at 350 degrees for 30 minutes.
6. Top with salsa.

The Raw Truth Recharge Zucchini Mexicali

Organic Ingredients
1 medium zucchini
1 medium onion
1 celery stalk
1 green pepper
1 shredded carrot
1 fresh garlic
¼ tsp. of basil
⅓ cup of taco sauce
2 medium tomatoes

Directions
1. Combine chopped vegetables in a skillet.
2. Cover and cook on medium-high for five minutes.
3. Stir in taco sauce, then cook five minutes more or until veggies are tender.

Zucchini Boats

Organic Ingredients
2 large zucchini
1 medium onion
1 fresh garlic – minced
1 red pepper
1 celery stalk
1 green pepper
1 medium carrot
1 large tomato

Directions:
1. Preheat oven to 300 degrees.
2. Slice zucchini in half. Use melon baller to scoop out leaving ¼ inch thickness. Boil water.
3. Put zucchini halves in boiling water for 1 minute.
4. Sauté garlic and onion. Add red peppers, the zucchini scooped out and chopped up, celery, green peppers, carrots, tomatoes. Sauté until soft.
5. Put mix into zucchini boats. Cover with simple sauce (below).
6. Cover boats with foil. Bake 30 to 40 minutes. After detox, you can sprinkle with a little Parmesan cheese for the last 5 minutes of bake time.

5-Minute Spaghetti Sauce:

Organic Ingredients
1 large can of tomato sauce
4 cans of diced or crushed tomatoes – no sugar added
2 large onions chopped
2-4 fresh garlic – minced
2 large red or green peppers chopped
¼ tsp. of Italian fresh spices (basil, oregano)

Directions
1. Sauté vegetables in 1 Tbsp. olive oil for 5 minutes on medium (avoid oil if detoxing).
2. Add tomato sauce and simmer for 30 minutes on low

Asian Lettuce Cups

Organic Ingredients
 1 ¼ lb organic ground turkey or soft non-gmo tofu
 1 Tbsp. olive oil
 1 clove garlic, minced
 1/8 tsp. ground ginger
 4 scallions
 1 can chopped water chestnuts
 12 Boston lettuce leaves
 3 Tbsp. hoisin sauce
 2 Tbsp. tamari
 1 Tbsp. rice vinegar
 2 tsp. roasted red chili paste
 1/8 tsp. salt

Directions
 1. Heat oil over medium heat. Add turkey, garlic, and ginger and cook until turkey is done. Stir until crumbled.
 2. Combine turkey or tofu mixture, onions, water chestnuts in a large bowl, stirring well, and set aside.
 3. In a small bowl, whisk together hoisin, soy sauce, rice vinegar, and chili paste and drizzle over the turkey mixture. Toss to coat completely.
 4. Add ¼ cup mixture to each lettuce leaf.

Sweet Potato Vegetable Lasagna

Ingredients
 Olive oil
 1 onion chopped
 1 small head of garlic, cloves chopped
 8 ounces fresh mushrooms
 2 carrots, chopped
 2 red bell peppers, chopped
 1 lb. silken tofu
 ½ teaspoon black pepper

1 teaspoon dried oregano
1 tsp. dried basil
1 tsp. dried rosemary
8 cups of marinara sauce
1-pound whole grain or spinach lasagna noodles (uncooked)
1 lb. fresh spinach
2 sweet potatoes, cooked and mashed (you can also use uncooked and cook lasagna longer)
6 Roma tomatoes, thinly sliced
1 cup raw cashews, ground

Directions

1. Set the oven at 400 degrees. Have on hand a 9-by-13-inch baking dish.
2. Add the olive oil to a large skillet and over a high heat cook the onion and garlic, stirring constantly, for 3 minutes. Add the mushrooms and cook, stirring often, for 5 minutes or until they release their liquid.
3. With a slotted spoon, transfer the vegetables to a large bowl, keeping the liquid in the pan.
4. In the same pan, cook the broccoli and carrots, stirring often, for 5 minutes. Add them to the mushroom mixture.
5. Drain the tofu by wrapping it in paper towels. Chop it into pieces. Add the tofu to the vegetables with the pepper, oregano, basil, and rosemary. Mix well.
6. Cover the bottom of the baking dish with a layer of sauce. Add a layer of noodles. Cover the noodles generously with sauce. Spread all the vegetables on top. Add another layer of noodles, then another layer of sauce.
7. Distribute all the spinach evenly on top. Use all the sweet potatoes to make another layer. Add sauce, then noodles, and finally more sauce. Lay the tomatoes on top.
8. Cover with foil and bake for 45 minutes.
9. Remove the foil. Sprinkle with cashews and return to the oven. Continue baking for 15 minutes. (Total baking time is 1 hour.) Let rest 15 minutes before serving.

Vegetable Quiche

Organic Ingredients
Olive oil
9 inch wheat, spelt or gluten free crust
Salt and pepper
Red pepper flakes
1 cup each of sweet onions, asparagus, red peppers, and mushrooms, chopped
4 eggs plus ½ cup of egg whites
1/3 cup of unsweetened almond milk

Directions
1. Preheat oven to 350 degrees.
2. Sauté vegetables using olive oil in a large frying pan for approximately 10 minutes; drain to reduce liquid.
3. Put veggies in the pie crust.
4. Beat eggs and whites until frothy.
5. Add the unsweetened almond milk
6. Add a couple dashes of red pepper flakes and mix thoroughly. Pour over the crust and veggies.
7. Bake at 350 degrees for approx. 20-30 minutes and enjoy!

Salads and Dressings

Sprouted Lentil Salad

Organic Ingredients
1 bag of dry lentils
6 organic carrots chopped or Julianne
6 organic celery stalks, chopped small
2 cups of walnuts
2 whole red peppers chopped small
2 cups of currants

Dressing Ingredients
1 level tsp. of cinnamon
1/8 tsp. of nutmeg
1 tsp. of Himalayan salt
¼ cup of balsamic vinegar
1 tsp. of Dijon mustard
¼ cup of olive oil
1 tsp. of coconut sugar (optional)

Directions
1. Soak the lentils overnight, then put in strainer and rinse them well twice a day for 3 days in strainer and allow to sprout.
2. After three days of sprouting, cook for 1 hour in enough water or vegetable broth to cover them in pan.
3. Bring to a boil on medium heat, drain, add carrots, celery, walnuts, and currants.
4. Once cooled, toss with dressing.

* Option: If short on time you can buy lentils already sprouted

Detox Salad Dressing

Organic Ingredients
½ cup of vinegar
1 tsp. of Dijon mustard
1/8 tsp. each of basil leaves, oregano, garlic, onion, pepper, paprika
½ cup of water

Directions
Whisk together thoroughly and enjoy!

Asian Salad

Organic Ingredients
2 cups of kale
2 cups Napa cabbage, shredded
1 red bell pepper, diced
2 scallions, sliced
½ cup grated carrot
1/3 cup sliced toasted almonds

Directions
1. Place all ingredients in salad bowl and toss with dressing below.

Dressing
⅓ cup unseasoned rice wine vinegar
¼ cup soy sauce or Bragg's Liquid Aminos
3 ½ Tbsp. raw honey
½ cup sesame oil
3 cloves garlic
1-½ inch piece of fresh ginger
1 Tbsp. organic natural peanut butter

Directions
1. Put all ingredients in a blender and blend until smooth.

Caesar Salad Dressing

Organic Ingredients
1 cup of olive oil
Juice from 3-4 lemons
5 cloves of garlic, pressed
Sea salt to taste
Fresh ground pepper
¼ cup of Parmesan cheese

Directions
1. Mix all ingredients by shaking in a closed container.
2. Serve over romaine lettuce.

Pear Walnut Salad

Organic Ingredients
2 cups of organic romaine lettuce or spring mix
2 Tbsp. of walnuts chopped
1 tsp. of extra virgin olive oil
1 Tbsp. balsamic vinegar
Add 2 sliced pears on top of salad and add dressing.

Quinoa Salad with Chickpeas, Feta and Apples

Organic Ingredients
One cup of quinoa, rinsed in a fine sieve
¼ cup of organic raisins
One 19 ounce (540 mL) can chickpeas, rinsed, boiled, and drained
One big handful of flat-leaf parsley, chopped
½ cup of low-fat crumbled feta (optional)
1 tart apple, chopped
½ cup of walnuts or almonds

Dressing

Shake ¼ cup of olive oil and ¼ cup balsamic vinegar together in a jar.

Directions

1. Cook 1 cup of quinoa according to package directions; dump into a wide salad bowl and set aside to cool. (Tip: add the raisins as it cools – the raisins will plump up as they absorb any excess moisture.)
2. Add the chickpeas, parsley, feta and apple and drizzle with dressing.
3. Toss, then sprinkle with toasted walnuts or almonds right before serving.

Spinach Salad

Organic Ingredients

10 oz. baby spinach
1 red bell pepper, diced
1 cucumber, sliced thin
1 small red onion, sliced
1 carrot, sliced thin
1 small head broccoli, cut small
1 cup almonds or pecans
Use organic ingredients. Place in and toss with balsamic dressing (below).

Balsamic Dressing:

Organic Ingredients
¼ sweet onion
¼ cup red wine vinegar
¼ cup of balsamic vinegar
2 Tbsp. fresh lemon juice
1 Tbsp. Dijon mustard
½ tsp. paprika
1 tsp. sea salt
1 cup of extra virgin olive oil

Directions
1. Blend first 3 ingredients in a blender.
2. Add the rest of the ingredients except for the oil.
3. Slowly add the oil.
4. Serve over the salad.

Summer Salad

Organic Ingredients
Organic spring mix and organic romaine hearts, cut in bite size pieces
Red bell pepper, diced
Broccoli, cut small
Clementines
Strawberries, sliced
Blueberries
Raspberries
Blackberries
Pecans
*Use as much as you need depending on how many servings you will need.

Directions
Toss ingredients in large bowl with strawberry poppyseed dressing (below).

Strawberry Poppyseed Dressing

Organic Ingredients
2 Tbsp. red wine vinegar
½ tsp. sea salt
½ tsp. dry ground mustard
½ cup extra virgin olive oil or walnut oil
1 cup organic strawberries
¼ tsp. poppyseeds

Directions
1. Blend first 4 ingredients in a blender.
2. Slowly add oil.
3. Stir in poppyseeds.

Sides

Delightful Sweet Potatoes

Organic Ingredients
4 large sweet potatoes
1 medium size butternut squash
½ cup apple cider
1 tsp. fresh grated nutmeg
½ tsp. cinnamon
The juice from ½ an orange
½ tsp. fresh orange zest

Directions
1. Preheat oven to 350 degrees.
2. In a 9x13 pan with 3 inches of water, bake the squash and sweet potatoes (be sure to pierce holes in them) at 350 degrees for 1½ hours.
3. Allow to cool, then scoop the squash and sweet potatoes from the skins, and discard along with the seeds.

4. Put the sweet potatoes and squash in a large bowl and use an electric mixer to beat until smooth.
5. Add the apple cider, nutmeg, cinnamon, orange juice, and orange zest.
6. Combine and put into a baking dish, bake at 350 degrees for 15 minutes or until heated through.

Almost Mashed Potatoes

Organic Ingredients
3 large, red potatoes, skins on
1 large turnip, peeled
½ head of cauliflower
1 tsp. garlic powder or fresh garlic
1 tsp. sea salt
½ tsp. black pepper
1 Tbsp. coconut oil
1 Tbsp. minced chives
1 tsp. minced rosemary

Directions
1. Chop veggies into about the same size. Add all of the vegetables in a large pot filled ¾ of the way with water and add the salt and garlic powder.
2. Boil until tender, around 20-30 minutes.
3. Strain and return to the pot, then add the butter, chives, rosemary, salt, and black pepper. Mash until the desired consistency.
(If you need to add some liquid you can add a couple tablespoons of veggie or chicken stock.)

3-5 Bean Salad

Organic Ingredients
1 can black beans
1 can of navy beans
1 can of chickpeas
2 large tomatoes
1 medium red onion
1 cucumber
1 yellow pepper
Handful of chopped parsley

Optional: jalapeño

Dressing
2 limes or lemons (optional)
1 Tbsp. cumin
½ cup oil
½ cup of Braggs Apple Cider Vinegar
Salt/pepper to taste

Directions
1. Cut and chop all ingredients in large bowl.
2. Pour dressing over ingredients and mix.
3. Let marinate in refrigerator for 1 hour before serving.

Quinoa with Garlic, Pine Nuts and Raisins

Organic Ingredients
1 cup of quinoa, rinsed well
¼ cup of pine nuts or sliced almonds
1 Tbsp. extra virgin olive oil
2 cloves garlic, thinly sliced
⅓ cup of chopped fresh parsley

¼ cup of raisins
1 Tbsp. of fresh lemon juice
Salt and pepper to taste

Directions

1. Place the quinoa in a saucepan and cook over medium heat until toasted, about 2 minutes. Add 1¾ cups of water or use low sodium veggie broth and bring to a boil.
2. Reduce the heat to medium-low and simmer, covered, until the liquid is absorbed, 10-15 minutes. Remove from the heat and let sit, covered about 2 minutes.
3. Meanwhile, toast pine nuts in a skillet over medium-high heat, stirring, until golden brown, about 3 minutes; transfer to plate.
4. Add the olive oil and garlic to the skillet and cook over medium-heat, stirring, until golden, about 2 minutes. Transfer the garlic, reserving the oil.
5. Fluff the quinoa with a fork. Add the pine nuts, garlic, reserved oil, parsley, raisins and lemon juice. Season with salt and pepper, and toss.

Dips, Spreads, and Dressings

Amazing Hummus

Organic Ingredients
1 (25oz.) can of organic chickpeas rinsed
½ cup organic baby spinach leaves (processed until finely chopped)
2 organic roasted red peppers
½ a can of artichokes
⅓ cup of tahini
¼ cup water
Juice from 1 lemon
1-2 cloves of garlic
¼ tsp. hot pepper flakes
½- 1 tsp. salt
1 tsp. ground cumin

Directions

Combine all ingredients in a food processor or Vitamix until smooth.

Bean Dip

Organic Ingredients

1 can black-eyed peas, rinsed
1 can black beans, rinsed
1 red bell pepper, diced
1 jalapeno pepper, diced
¼ cup diced red onion
1 cup celery, diced small

Marinade Ingredients

¾ cup extra virgin olive oil
½ cup apple cider vinegar

Directions

1. Place peas, beans, peppers, onion and celery in bowl.
2. Heat marinade ingredients in a saucepan until sugar is dissolved. Do not bring to a boil.
3. Allow marinade to cool, then pour over bean/vegetable mixture.
4. Refrigerate overnight. Serve with healthy chips.

Guacamole

Ingredients

4 ripe avocados, peeled and pitted
2 lemons, juiced
2 tsp. minced garlic
1 tomato, diced
¼ cup cilantro, chopped
¼ cup diced red onion

¼ tsp. ground cumin
5 jalapeño chilies, minced; 3 of the chilies seeded
Salt and chili powder to taste

Directions
1. In a large bowl, coarsely mash avocados and combine with lemon juice.
2. Add the remaining ingredients to the avocado mixture, stirring until combined.
3. Refrigerate for 30 minutes and serve.

*Large avocadoes are recommended for this recipe. A large avocado averages about 8 ounces. If using smaller or larger size avocadoes, adjust the quantity accordingly.

Vegetable Dip

Organic Ingredients
4 garlic cloves, minced and then mashed
2 fifteen-ounce cans of garbanzo beans (chickpeas), drained and rinsed
⅔ cup of tahini
⅓ cup of fresh squeezed lemon juice
½ cup of water
¼ cup of olive oil
½ teaspoon of salt
1 fresh red pepper, chopped

Directions
1. In a food processor, combine the mashed garlic, garbanzo beans, lemon juice, ½ cup of water and olive oil. Process until smooth.
2. Add salt, starting at a half a teaspoon, to taste.
3. Add red pepper.
4. Spoon into serving dish and sprinkle with chopped parsley.

Smoothies

For all smoothies, place ingredients in Vitamix, NutriBullet or other powerful blender.

Powershot Green Smoothie

Ingredients
1 tsp. of powershot Raw Organic Greens
    8 oz of coconut milk
    1 Tbsp. of chia seeds
    ½ cup of ice

Chocolate Peanut Butter Frozen Smoothie

Organic Ingredients
    2 bananas, peeled and cut in slices and frozen
    1 cup unsweetened vanilla almond milk
    ¼ cup powdered organic peanut butter
    ⅛ cup raw cacao powder

Peanut Butter and Chocolate Protein Smoothie

Ingredients
    6-8 ounces of unsweetened almond milk
    2 Tbsp. of powdered organic peanut or almond butter
    1 tsp. of raw cacao
    1 frozen banana and some ice
    Scoop of plant-based protein powder

Green Smoothie #1

Organic Ingredients
    3 Tbsp. plant protein powder (optional)
    2-inch piece of ginger (peeled if not organic)

2 cups of leafy greens (kale, collards, romaine, spinach, chard)
1 cup of celery
1 frozen banana
¼ cup of mixed fresh or frozen organic berries of your choice
(strawberries, blueberries, cranberries)
½ cup filtered water

Green Smoothie #2

Organic Ingredients
　1 bunch organic dark kale
　½ bunch organic celery
　½ bunch cilantro or parsley
　1 organic cucumber with ends removed
　1 lemon with peel removed
　2 inches of fresh ginger root
　1 organic apple
　1 organic carrot
　1 cup water

Sunrise Green Smoothie

Organic Ingredients
　4 cups spinach
　1 cucumber, diced
　½ cup water
　1 lemon or lime, juiced
　4 carrots, peeled and diced
　¼ cup of strawberries/Blueberries/blackberries
　1 cup of ice (optional)
　1 Tbsp. chia seeds

Snacks

Kale Chips
Remember kale is considered to be a highly nutritious vegetable with powerful antioxidant properties; kale is high in beta-carotene, vitamins K and C and calcium, and is considered to be anti-inflammatory.

Organic Ingredients
One bunch kale
Olive or coconut oil
Sea salt (optional)

Directions
1. Preheat oven to 300 degrees.
2. Cut the stems off the kale, wash, and thoroughly dry.
3. Put on baking pan lined with parchment paper, drizzle with olive oil (optional) and sprinkle with sea salt.
4. Bake for 20-25 minutes until dry and crunchy.

Roasted Chick Peas

Organic Ingredients
1 (12 ounce) can of chickpeas (garbanzo beans), drained
2 Tbsp. olive oil
Salt (optional)
Garlic salt (optional)
Pepper (optional)
Dash of rosemary

Directions
1. Preheat oven to 450 degrees F.
2. Blot chickpeas with a paper towel to dry them.
3. In a bowl, toss chickpeas with olive oil, and season to taste with salt, garlic salt, and cayenne pepper, if using.
4. Spread on a baking sheet, and bake for 30 to 40 minutes, until browned and crunchy. Watch carefully the last few minutes to avoid burning.

Sprouted Grain Tortilla Chips

Organic Ingredient
1 package of Sprouted Grain Ezekiel tortilla wraps

Directions
1. Preheat oven to 350 degrees.
2. Place wraps on cookie sheet.
3. Bake for seven minutes, longer if you want them crispy.
4. Break up into pieces and dip in your favorite bean, hummus, salsa or avocado dip!

Soups and Stews

Minestrone Quinoa Soup

Organic Ingredients
2 Tbsp. olive oil, best quality
1 cup of diced carrots
1 cup of diced fennel
1 cup of diced red onion
1 celery rib, diced
2 zucchini diced
4 cloves garlic, minced
2 bay leaves
2 tsp. thyme, chopped
6 cups of vegetable broth
1 ½ cups cannellini beans, cooked
2 cups seeded and diced plum tomatoes
½ cup quinoa, rinsed
Salt and pepper
1 cup spinach, fresh and finely chopped
2 Tbsp. basil, sliced
½ cup Parmesan cheese, grated

Directions
1. Heat olive oil in a heavy stock pot over medium heat. Add carrots, fennel, onion, celery garlic, bay leaves and thyme and cook for 5 minutes. Add zucchini and cook for an additional 4 minutes.
2. Add broth, beans, tomatoes and quinoa. Increase the heat to bring to a boil. Reduce to low and simmer for 20 minutes or until the quinoa is tender.
3. Remove bay leaves and sprinkle with salt and pepper.
4. Stir in spinach and basil just before serving.

Minestrone Vegetable Soup

Organic Ingredients
3 cups each of carrots, celery, zucchini, onion
1 bag of dry great northern beans soaked and cooked or 3 cans of beans
Two 28-ounce cans diced tomatoes in juice
Three 32-ounce containers of organic vegetable broth
12 fresh basil leaves
4 cloves of garlic
1 Tbsp. fresh rosemary
1 Tbsp. Himalayan salt
pepper to taste

Directions:
1. Cook celery, carrots, zucchini in one tablespoon of olive oil for 5 minutes on high. Add vegetable broth tomatoes, and beans. Cook until vegetables are tender but not soft.
2. Make pesto with basil leaves cut very small, minced garlic cloves, and rosemary mixed together with one teaspoon olive oil and add to soup the last 5 minutes of cooking. The fresh pesto is what makes the difference so don't skip this step.
(For Detox, omit oil and beans).

Black Bean Chili

Organic Ingredients
1 Tbsp. extra virgin olive oil
½ cup celery, diced
½ cup onion, diced
½ cup carrot, diced
1 clove garlic, minced
¾ tsp. cumin

14-ounce can diced tomatoes with green chilies
3 cans black beans, drained and rinsed
3 ⅔ cups organic low-sodium chicken broth or vegetable broth
1 cup mild organic salsa

Directions
1. Heat oil in saucepan. Add celery, onion and carrots.
2. Cook until soft, about 10 minutes.
3. Add garlic. Cook another minute.
4. Stir in beans, broth, tomatoes, and salsa. Simmer uncovered for 15 minutes.

Cream of Tomato Soup

Organic Ingredients
3 Tbsp. extra-virgin olive oil
½ cup chopped red onion
2 tsp. minced garlic
1/4 tsp. red pepper flakes
2 28-ounce cans organic whole tomatoes in juice
3 cups organic low-sodium chicken broth
½ tsp. sea salt
¼ tsp. ground black pepper
⅓ cup chopped fresh basil leaves
⅓ cup unsweetened almond milk

Directions
1. In medium saucepan, sauté onion and garlic in oil over medium heat until soft, approximately 5 minutes.
2. Add tomatoes, pepper flakes and chicken broth and bring to a boil over medium-high heat. Boil for 25 minutes.
3. Add sea salt and pepper.
4. Remove from heat.
5. Using hand blender, blend slightly. Stir in basil leaves and almond milk.

Curried Butternut and Red Lentil Soup with Spinach

Organic Ingredients
1 Tbsp. olive oil
1 medium onion, chopped
1 medium butternut squash, peeled and diced
1 garlic clove, minced
1 Tbsp. minced fresh ginger
1 Tbsp. hot or mild curry powder
One dash of cinnamon
1 14.5-ounce can crushed tomatoes
1 cup red lentils, picked over, rinsed, and drained
5 cups vegetable broth
Salt and freshly ground black pepper
3 cups chopped spinach

Directions
1. In a large soup pot, heat the oil over medium heat. Add the onion, squash, and garlic.
2. Cover and cook until softened, about 10 minutes.
3. Stir in the ginger and curry powder, and then add the tomatoes, lentils, broth, and salt and pepper to taste. Bring to boil, and then reduce heat to low and simmer, uncovered, until the lentils and vegetables are tender, stirring occasionally, about 45 minutes.
4. About 15 minutes before serving, stir in the chard or kale.
5. Taste, adjusting seasonings if necessary, and serve.

Curried Sweet Potato and Chickpea Stew

Organic Ingredients
1 ½ Tbsp. olive oil
1 ½ cups thinly sliced onion
2 cups coarsely chopped green bell pepper
1 ½ Tbsp. curry powder

½ Tbsp. cumin
½ tsp. salt, divided
1 quart of low-sodium vegetable broth
4 cups peeled ½-inch pieces of sweet potato or butternut squash
1 can (19 oz.) unsalted chickpeas, drained and rinsed
1 cup light unsweetened coconut milk
¼ cup finely chopped cilantro
⅜ tsp. ground black pepper

Directions

1. Heat oil in a large stockpot or Dutch oven over medium heat. Stir in onion and bell pepper; cook for 8 minutes or until tender.
2. Stir in curry powder, cumin, and ¼ teaspoon salt; cook for 2 minutes.
3. Add vegetable broth and sweet potatoes and bring to a boil; reduce heat, cover, and simmer for 15 minutes or until potatoes are tender.
4. Remove 1 cup of sweet potatoes and mash with a fork. Stir mashed potatoes back into pot and bring to a boil; reduce heat and boil gently for 5 minutes to allow mixture to thicken.
5. Stir in chickpeas, coconut milk, cilantro, and black pepper. Cook for 1 to 2 minutes or until warm throughout.
6. Stir in remaining ¼ teaspoon salt (optional) and serve.

Lentil, Coconut and Wilted Spinach Soup

Organic Ingredients
⅔ cup of lentils, rinsed
4 cups of organic vegetable stock
1 large chopped onion
2 fat cloves of garlic chopped
2 tsp. of ground cumin
1 cup of canned coconut milk
2-3 Tbsp. of Braggs Aminos
4 handfuls of baby spinach, (about 2 cups)
Kosher salt and fresh ground black pepper

Directions
1. Put lentils in a large saucepan and add enough cold water just to cover.
2. Boil lentils for 10 minutes, then add the remaining ingredients, except the spinach.
3. Reduce the heat and simmer for 20-30 minutes or until the lentils are tender.
4. Put a small handful of spinach in the bowls and ladle the hot soup on top.

Pumpkin Coconut Soup

Organic Ingredients
1 Tbsp. coconut oil
1 medium white onion, diced
½ tsp. of ground cinnamon
½ tsp. of chili powder
½ tsp. of cumin
Pinch ground nutmeg
3 cups of low-sodium chicken broth or veggie broth
3 cups of pumpkin puree (or squash or sweet potato)
1 Tbsp. fresh lime juice
1 cup of light coconut milk
Sea salt and ground black pepper to taste
¾ cup of nonfat plain Greek yogurt
6 Tbsp. raw pumpkin seeds

Directions
1. Heat oil in large saucepan on medium high. Add onion and cook, stirring frequently, until softened and translucent, about 5 minutes.
2. Add cinnamon, chili powder, cumin, and nutmeg and cook for about 1 minute, stirring frequently, until fragrant.

3. Add broth and pumpkin and whisk until incorporated and smooth, adding up to one cup of water if broth is too thick.
4. Bring to boil, reduce heat to medium-low and simmer for 5 minutes, stirring frequently.
5. Remove from heat and add lime juice. Stir in coconut milk and season with salt and pepper.
6. Top each serving of soup with 2 Tbsp. yogurt and 1 Tbsp. pumpkin seeds.

The Raw Truth Recharge Detox Soup

Organic Ingredients
3-4 cartons of organic vegetable stock
Fill with chopped vegetables:
2 minced garlic cloves
2 small onions, diced
4 diced carrots
4 diced tomatoes
2 zucchini
4 celery stalks
½ cup of purple cabbage chopped
1 cup of squash green beans
Add Spices – 1 tsp. of basil, oregano, and parsley
Pepper to taste.
1 cup spinach or kale (add at end)

Directions
1. Add together all ingredients at once except spinach or kale.
2. Bring to boil, then simmer on low for 30 minutes. At the 25-minute mark, add the spinach or kale.

Note: After Detox you can sauté the onions, garlic, celery and carrots first in a little EVOO, and later add beans, legumes, chickpeas etc. You can also add in other organic vegetables of your choice.

Shrimp Coconut Spinach/Kale Soup

Organic Ingredients
1 Tbsp. of extra virgin olive oil (cold pressed is best)
1 16-ounce package of organic spinach or kale (either works great)
1 can of low-fat coconut milk
1 32-ounce carton of Thai culinary stock (found near vegetable broth)
1 16-ounce package (36-40 count) of peeled cooked shrimp, thawed
2 ½ Tbsp. of Bragg's Aminos
Salt and pepper to taste

Directions
1. Add oil and spinach to a stockpot and cook on medium, stirring, for 3-4 minutes.
2. Add coconut milk and stock; bring to simmer on medium-high, about 5 minutes.
3. Stir in shrimp. Cover and remove from heat. Let stand about 5 minutes.
4. Stir in liquid Aminos or soy sauce and season to taste.

Vegan Lentil Soup

Organic Ingredients
1 Tbsp. of Olive oil or Vegetable Broth
3 chopped carrots
6 chopped celery stalks
1 medium yellow onions or 1 large
2 cloves of garlic chopped
2 cartons of vegetable broth or 4 cups
2 cups of sprouted Lentils
28 ounces of diced tomatoes
1 cup of water
1 cup of fresh spinach chopped
1 Tbsp. of lemon juice (approx. ½ lemon)
1 tsp. salt

1 tsp. of pepper
1 tsp. cumin
1 tsp. of dried thyme

Directions
1) Place a large pot on stove and add cooking oil or vegetable broth. Cook onions, carrots, celery under tender.
2) Add all other ingredients, (except spinach and lemon juice which you will add at the end.). Turn all other ingredients in pan on high and bring soup to boil.
3) Turn soup down to simmer for 25-30 minutes. Add lemon juice and spinach to soup and allow greens to wilt. Enjoy!
4) Eat and store leftover soup for 5 days or freeze in contains up to three months.

Mediterranean Fish

Organic Ingredients
1 cup summer squash
1 cup zucchini
½ red onion sliced thin
2 pounds of cod or another whitefish
1 cup of yellow and red bell pepper
¼ cup roasted red pepper, plus 1 Tbsp. liquid
¼ cup artichokes quartered plus 2 Tbsp. liquid
¼ cup feta cheese
2 Tbsp. extra virgin olive oil
1 clove of garlic, minced
Juice of 1 lemon
½ tsp. salt
1 tsp. rosemary

Directions

1. Preheat oven to 375 degrees.
2. Drizzle olive oil on the bottom of a 9x13 pan, then layer zucchini, summer squash, roasted red pepper, and artichokes on the bottom of the pan.
3. Sprinkle of the half-teaspoon of salt over the veggies.
4. Layer the fish, drizzle with artichoke juice and roasted red pepper liquid, sprinkle with salt and chopped rosemary, fresh squeezed lemon juice, and a clove of minced garlic.
5. Spread the bell peppers and red onion and feta cheese over the top of the fish.
6. Bake at 375 degrees for 30 minutes.

Vegetable Stew

Organic Ingredients

1 carton low-sodium vegetable broth
¼ cup chopped onion
1 small organic zucchini, sliced
2 large organic carrots, washed and sliced
1 clove garlic, minced
1 red bell pepper, diced
2 organic stalks celery, sliced
1 cup organic broccoli, cut in small pieces
1 cup organic cauliflower, cut in small pieces
1 15-ounce. can organic fire-roasted diced tomatoes
¼ cup fresh basil leaves or 1 tsp. dried basil
1 jar organic marinara sauce (no sugar added)

Directions

1. Place all ingredients except marinara sauce in a large soup pot and bring to a boil.
2. Turn down heat to medium-high and cook until vegetables are tender.
3. Add marinara sauce and heat on low for 30 minutes.

Desserts

Banana Split Milkshake

Organic Ingredients
1 cup plain unsweetened non-dairy frozen yogurt
½ cup unsweetened vanilla almond milk
2 bananas, peeled
1 cup frozen organic strawberries
½ cup pineapple (fresh or canned)
scoop of vanilla protein powder

Directions
Place in Vitamix and blend on high until smooth.

Blueberry Banana Ginger "Ice Cream"

Organic Ingredients
1 frozen banana
½ cup fresh blueberries or strawberries
½ Tbsp. fresh ginger, minced
One dash of cinnamon

Directions
Place all the ingredients into a high speed blender or Vitamix and blend until just combined. If it's too thick, you can add a little coconut or almond milk.

Ice Cream Pumpkin Pie

Organic Crust Ingredients
1 cup roasted pecans, coarsely chopped
2 Tbsp. melted coconut oil
½ tsp. coconut sugar

Crust Directions
1. Mix all ingredients well in a small bowl.
2. Lightly grease bottom of pie plate with coconut oil or cooking spray.
3. Pat mixture on bottom of pie plate (You can double the recipe if you want to go up the sides of your pie plate).
4. Put crust in freezer.

Filling Ingredients
2 cups unsweetened plain non-dairy frozen yogurt slightly softened
1 cup canned pumpkin
½ cup coconut sugar
½ tsp. fine sea salt
¾ tsp. pumpkin pie spice or ¼ tsp. each of cinnamon, nutmeg and ginger
3 cans coconut milk
3-4 drops pure liquid vanilla stevia

*One day before making your pie, put all 3 cans of coconut milk in your refrigerator.

Directions
1. In a bowl, blend canned pumpkin, coconut sugar, sea salt, and pumpkin pie spice with an electric mixer on medium speed until well-blended.
2. Take out two cans of unsweetened coconut milk from your fridge. After sitting overnight, it will separate. Open cans and scoop out the solid milk (don't use the liquid in the cans) with a spoon and place in a small mixing bowl.
3. Using an electric mixer, beat milk on medium speed until it looks like whipped cream. Fold it into your pumpkin mixture w/ a rubber spatula until blended.
4. Remove your pie crust from the freezer. It should be hardened.
5. Spread the 2 cups of vanilla frozen dessert on top of your crust. Place in freezer until hardened, at least half an hour.
6. Put pumpkin mixture on top of vanilla frozen dessert. Return to freezer until hardened.

7. Take the last can of coconut milk from the refrigerator and whip the solid milk with 3 or 4 drops of pure vanilla stevia until it looks like whipped cream.
8. Place whipped mixture on top of pumpkin pie and place in the freezer for 15 minutes or until ready to serve.

Bake Peanut Butter Cookies

Organic Ingredients
½ cup coconut oil
½ cup raw cacao powder
¾ cup coconut sugar
½ cup unsweetened almond milk
½ tsp. vanilla extract
½ cup organic natural peanut butter
1 ½ cups gluten-free quick cooking oats
1 cup unsweetened coconut
½ cup roasted pecans

Directions
1. Preheat oven to 350 degrees.
2. Boil coconut oil, cacao powder, coconut sugar and almond milk in a small saucepan for 1 minute. Turn off heat.
3. Add vanilla extract, peanut butter, oats, coconut and pecans.
4. Place on cookie sheet and bake at 350 degrees for about 8-9 minutes, turning once.
5. Drop by tablespoons onto a piece of waxed paper and let cool.
6. Store in covered container or gallon-size Ziploc bag.

Gluten-Free Almond Oat Chocolate Chip Cookie

Organic Ingredients
2 ½ cups almond meal
*½ cup gluten-free oat flour
2 Tbsp. coconut flour

1 tsp. baking soda

¼ tsp. sea salt

½ cup coconut palm sugar

½ cup coconut oil

2 pastured eggs

1 tsp. vanilla extract

½ cup 70% raw chocolate chips or cacao nibs

Directions

1. Preheat oven to 375 degrees.
2. Combine almond meal, oat flour, coconut flour, sugar, soda, and salt.
3. In a separate bowl, beat coconut oil, eggs and vanilla together. Mix the wet ingredients with the dry ingredients, than fold in the chocolate chips.
4. Drop the batter by spoonsful onto a cookie sheet lined with parchment paper.
5. Bake for 10 minutes.

* To make grain free use ground flax seeds in place of oat flour

Chocolate Mousse

Organic Ingredients

2 ripe avocadoes

¼ cup of raw cacao powder

¼ cup of coconut nectar

¼ cup of unsweetened almond milk

1 tsp. of vanilla

Directions

1. Mix all ingredients in Vitamix or mixer and pour into cups or gluten-free graham cracker crust.

Cranberry Pecan Banana Muffins

Organic Ingredients
2 ripe bananas
1½ cups sprouted wheat flour
¾ cup coconut sugar
2 tsp. baking powder
1 tsp. baking soda
2 eggs
1 tsp. salt
¼ cup dried cranberries, or fresh chopped
⅓ cup coconut oil, melted
2 Tbsp. chopped pecans

Directions
1. Preheat oven to 350 degrees.
2. Mash the bananas with a fork or potato masher, then stir in xylitol, eggs, flour, baking powder, baking soda, salt, and coconut oil.
3. Mix until combined then add the pecans and cranberries.
4. Fill a lightly greased muffin pan ½ way and bake 20 to 30 minutes at 350 degrees.

Peanut Butter Protein Bars

Organic Ingredients
½ cup steel-cut oatmeal flour (put ½ c oats in a blender and process)
½ cup almond flour
½ cup plant-based vanilla protein powder
½ cup applesauce unsweetened
½ cup water
¼ cup date honey (8 medjool dates, pitted boil until soft in ½ cup water about 5 min puree in food processor or Vitamix)
1 Tbsp. each of ground flax seeds, peanut butter powder, chia seeds
½ tsp. salt
½ cup of raw cacao nibs
½ cup of unsweetened coconut flakes

Directions

1. Use a cookie scoop and place scoops of batter in the freezer for a frozen cookie dough treat, OR
2. Bake in a 9x9 pan spritzed with EVOO and bake at 350 degrees for 20-30 min.

Coconut No Bake Cookies

Organic Ingredients

½ cup all natural peanut butter
1/3 cup coconut nectar
½ cup coconut oil
2 Tbsp. cacao powder
½ cup large unsweetened coconut flakes
1 tsp. vanilla extract
2 cups old-fashioned oats or steel-cut oats

Directions

1. Heat the peanut butter, coconut nectar, coconut oil and cacao powder on medium heat until it melts and comes to a boil.
2. Remove from the heat and add oatmeal, coconut flakes, and vanilla.
3. Transfer to a bar pan and let cool before cutting and serving.

Black Bean Brownies

Organic Ingredients

28-ounce can of organic black beans
2 eggs
¾ cup coconut sugar
⅓ cup coconut oil
¼ cup cacao powder
¼ cup water
1 tsp. salt
1 tsp. baking soda
1 tsp. vanilla extract
½ tsp. cinnamon

Directions
1. Preheat oven to 350 degrees.
2. Put all of the ingredients in a Vitamix or food processor and blend until smooth.
3. Pour into a lightly greased 9x13 pan and bake for 15 to 30 minutes at 350 degrees.

Mint Chocolate Bombs

Ingredients
¼ cup coconut oil
½ cup coconut butter
¼ cup cacao powder 2 Tbsp. coconut flour
2 Tbsp. monk fruit sweetener 10 drops of mint oil

Directions
1. Place the coconut oil and coconut butter in a small pan and melt over low heat.
2. Add in all the other ingredients and whisk until well incorporated.
3. Place about 1 Tbsp. of the melted mixture into a silicon mould pan and place in the fridge until it firms up (approx an hour).
4. Remove from the mould when it sets and place in an airtight container in the fridge
5. If you don't like mint, skip it and you can use vanilla extract or any other flavor of your choosing.

Notes
You will want to place the silicon pan on a tray before you begin to fill it up so the mixture doesn't spill all over the place given that these silicon trays are usually quite flimsy.

No Bake Pumpkin Pie (Gluten Free, Vegan)
An easy NO BAKE pumpkin pie that is delicious and takes no time to whip up!

Serves: 1 pie

Ingredients Crust
1.5 cup of raw almonds 1 cup of pecans
15 dates neglet noor or 6 medjool 2 Tbsp. coconut nectar
2 Tbsp. coconut oil

Filling
- 2.5 cups of pumpkin puree
- 1 can coconut cream (the fatty part only, liquid discarded)
- 1 cup of coconut sugar
- 1½ tsp. cinnamon
- grated nutmeg to taste
- pinch of salt
- 1 Tbsp. of agar agar (MUST ingredient)

Directions Crust
1. Lightly toast almonds and pecans (approx. 30 minutes) in 250 oven checking frequently to make sure they toast evenly. You'll want them lightly toasted and you'll know they're done when they begin smell aromatic.
2. Meanwhile, place pitted dates in food processor and process until smooth. If the dates are quite hard, you can place them in hot water for a few minutes to soften them up. Then strain, squeeze out the excess water and place in a food processor. Place the pureed dates in a shallow pot and add in coconut oil and coconut nectar. Warm over medium heat until the coconut oil melts and the mixture becomes a nice paste.
3. Once the nuts have cooled. Place in a food processor and pulse until the mixture is coarsely ground to your desired consistency. I like mine coarse, as I like to texture of the larger pieces of nuts. Stir the pulsed nuts into the pasty date mixture. Stir until well combined. Place in a pie dish and pat down until firmly pressed at the bottom of the pan. You can use parchment paper or waxed paper to help you flatten it out without having the mixture stick to your hands.

Filling
1. Place pumpkin puree in a deep pot. Add to this the cream from one can of full fat coconut cream. Discard the liquid and only use the creamy part of the canned product. Refrigerating the can ahead of time can help with this. Add the sugar, cinnamon, nutmeg and sea salt.
2. Bring to a boil over medium/high heat, stirring frequently. Then add in the agar agar and allow it to boil for another minute, stirring periodically. The agar agar can't be skipped! It's the key ingredient to thicken the pie and allow it to set.
3. Place the boiled mixture over the pressed down crust and refrigerate immediately. Refrigerate for a minimum of 3 hours and then serve.
4. I like to prepare this a day in advance so it has plenty of time to set.

Chocolate cake

Ingredients
3 cups of light spelt flour or gluten free flour blend
½ cup of cacao powder 1 teaspoon baking soda
1⅓ cup of unsweetened apple sauce 1½ cups of coconut sugar
¾ cup of warm water
¾ cup of cashew mylk (home made preferred)
⅓ cup avocado oil
1 Tbsp. apple cider vinegar
1 tsp. vanilla
⅓ cup of dark chocolate chips

Directions
1. Preheat oven to 350 on bake setting. Grease a 10 inch pan or a medium sized bundt pan and set aside.
2. Place flour into large bowl, add to it the cacao power and baking soda. Whisk for a couple of minutes to ensure well incorporated.
3. Place apple sauce, coconut sugar, water, mylk, oil, vinegar and vanilla into a blender and blend for a minute until completely smooth.

4. Make a well in the center of the dry ingredients and pour the wet mixture in. Fold or whisk until fully incorporated by hand. Try not to over-mix, but ensure no flour is visible.
5. Next gently fold in the chocolate chips.
6. Pour the mixture into the pan and place in the oven. Bake for 25 minutes or until a toothpick comes out clean. It may take longer than 25 minutes depending on your oven, however be certain to not over-bake, otherwise the cake will turn out too dry.

Notes
To make the apple sauce yourself, cut up a few apples into small cubes, measuring two cupfuls, discarding the peel and core. Place into a small pot, add 2 tablespoons of water to this and cover and cook for 5-7 minutes until the apples are tender. You can then just add this directly to the blender and blend with the rest of the ingredients.

Grain Free Banana Bread

Makes 1 loaf

Ingredients
4 large Organic Eggs
2 Tbsp. of coconut oil melted (plus more for greasing)
1 tsp. of pure vanilla extract
3 Tbsp. of coconut nectar (or raw honey)
½ tsp. of apple cider vinegar
¼ cup of almond flour
½ cup of coconut flour
1tsp. of baking soda
½ tsp. of Redmond real salt
3 large ripe bananas
½ cup of coconut milk
¼ cup of chopped walnuts, chocolate chips, dried fruit or raisins optional.

Directions

1. Preheat oven to 350 F
2. Grease sides and bottom of an 8 and ½ by 4 and ½ inch loaf pan.
3. Combine most of the wet ingredients, coconut nectar, 2 Tbsp. of melted coconut oil, eggs, vanilla and apple cider vinegar in a bowl and beat on high for 40 seconds.
4. Combine the dry ingredients, almond flour, coconut flour, baking soda and salt in a bowl and add the to the wet ingredients.
5. Mash the bananas and add coconut milk in a bowl. Beat on Medium until mixed
6. Mix in walnuts or any of the optional ingredients.
7. Pour the batter into the greased loaf pan and bake for 40 minutes or until an inserted tooth pick to the middle comes out clean.
8. Remove from oven and coo for 15 minutes before slicing.

Summary:

If you don't make deliberate decisions in your life to do the things to feed your mind, body, soul, spirit – they won't happen. You need to make time to pray every morning/night and do devotions. Make time to exercise, prepare your healthy food, brush your teeth, care for your family, spend time with your children and spouse or significant other, clean, prepare your meals, cook, work, go to your health checkups, pray, read, think, and sleep 8 hours. That's a lot of stuff to do in 24 hours and get work in on top of it. We have to prioritize each day and remember our time with God must be number one in our life. I take my supplements and drink my warm water and lemon while I'm spending time with God in the morning, and I do it without fail.

People tell me they don't have time to do this or that. Don't have time to work out or do any of the things I mentioned? I don't either, but I make time. We all have the same amount of time in the day. It's what you do with that time that's your choice and makes a difference in your life. Prioritize. Get up early or do what you have to do to fit the important stuff in. Make the choice to pray, do devotions, worship, and be fed spiritually every day every way you can as if your life depends on it because it does.

I promise you, God will bless you for that a thousand times over for making HIM a priority.

Proverbs 4:20-22 says *"My son, pay attention to what I say; listen closely to my works. Do not let them out of your sight, keep them within your heart; for they are the life for those who find them and health to a man's whole body."*

My life verse:

"Trust in the Lord with all your Heart and lean not on your own understanding; in all your ways acknowledge Him and He will make your paths straight."
Proverbs 3:5-6

My life and death verse:

John 3:16 – "For God so loved the world that He gave His only begotten Son, that whoever believes in Him shall not perish, but have eternal life."

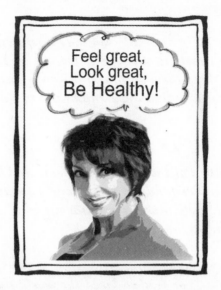

TESTIMONIALS AND ENDORSEMENTS

What Others Have Said About Robbie and The Raw Truth Recharge

I've struggled with my weight my entire life. I was on my first diet in the fourth grade. That diet marked the beginning of my yo-yo dieting journey. Over the years I've developed the worst habits and could never stick to anything long enough to lose the weight. It wasn't until I gave my life back to the Lord that things started to change. I remember praying out to God asking for help and for Him to "show" me what diet to follow. I figured since everything else was in the Bible, He would have a diet in there as well. One night, I was very depressed, lying on my couch. I was listening to a message from Charles Stanley, and he mentioned Proverbs 3:5. I got up and grabbed my Bible to read what I had just heard. It read, "Trust in the LORD with all your heart and lean not on your own understanding; in all your ways submit to Him, and He will make your paths straight. Do not be wise in your own eyes; fear the LORD and shun evil. *This will bring health to your body and nourishment to your bones.*"

At that moment I realized I needed to hand this issue over to Him. I got on my knees and asked God to enter in to help me be released from my addiction to food. He showed me that it was more than just my physical appearance but more about where my heart was. I chose food over everything. It was my crutch in life. In order for me to "fix" the problem, I had to put God first in my life. I had to choose God over the cupcake when I was having an emotional breakdown, or the bag of chips when I was overwhelmed with anxiety.

He also brought me the best person to help me through it all. Robbie Raugh not only became my coach, but my accountability partner and friend. She taught me how to heal my body from the inside out. I relearned how to eat, how to exercise, and how to pull God right in when things got tough. Now, it's more about being healthy so that I am able to do the things God has called me to do. I am so grateful for Robbie and her devotion to helping change people and their health. She is one of the most important people in my life, and I am beyond blessed to have her in my corner rooting for me!

—**Keri Cardinale**
Radio Host of "The Keri and Robbie Show" WDCX 99.5FM

Robbie,

I will never forget the first time that we met. It actually was a day that I was fearful of. Not of you, but to face the truth about what my life had consisted of. But little did I realize that you were not to be "feared" but you were someone that brought great peace and a greater purpose to my life. You made clear and somewhat easy for me to understand what would make me healthy and literally participated in saving my life. You gave me the insight and helped with the challenges that I faced all of my life. As a child I grew up in a very dysfunctional home where eating for us was the only solace we could ever experience. But you helped me to understand beyond that into what healthy eating could produce. And when I stood on those scales last year at Kingdom Bound, having lost a total of sixty-five pounds, I knew my life would never be the same. And it has not.

Love you much Robbie! I'm going for it all!

—**Pastor Marty Macdonald**
City Church
Batavia, NY 14020
www.TheCityChurch.com

There are many reasons why I decided to join Robbie and the Raw Truth Recharge for our four-month journey. I knew I needed to lose weight and get in shape, but the ultimate reason for me was my battle with high blood pressure and borderline diabetes. My blood sugar numbers were getting way too high, and I wasn't feeling the way I knew I should. It only took a few weeks of eating healthy and exercising that I saw all my numbers dropping significantly. Again, the number that was really most exciting for me was my blood sugar, which had gotten as high as 180 at one point before I started. During the four months I saw that number consistently staying on or below 100! To God be the glory!

It is a daily battle for me to continue to do the things I know I MUST do in the areas of eating healthy and exercising, but I thank Robbie and God most of all for the education I got in how important it is to take care of this body God has given me.

I highly encourage and challenge anyone to join Robbie on this journey to take care of your "mobile home"—God's way!

—**Pastor Matt Gold**
Alden Community Church

I was broken. Hope was lost! But God had the day as He always does. "Trust in the Lord with all your heart...Proverbs 3:5a...then you will have healing for your body and strength for your bones" Proverbs 3:8 NLT.

I had heard of the Raw Truth Recharge on WDCX and, ever the skeptic, felt it was bunk, even though I knew of some people it had helped. At Kingdom Bound Festival 2014, there were Raw Truth seminars to attend, and I was very much set against going. I could do this on my own, even though I've tried other "diets" in the past, but…God had a plan. He drew my wife Laurie— who can be persuasive—and me to the WDCX tent on Monday to hear Robbie. The passion, conviction and knowledge with which Robbie spoke hit me hard, and brought us back Tuesday and again on Wednesday. Robbie took time to speak to us afterward each day and encouraged us to attend an upcoming seminar. Our discussions were emotional as she saw the pain of lost hope and our being, as Robbie says, "Sick and thick and tired!"

We attended the seminar and enrolled in the Recharge…WOW… a commitment! But…the Raw Truth Recharge has changed our family's lives. Through the Recharge Protocol I've lost over sixty six pounds, over eight inches from my waist and my body fat has decreased more than twelve points…over 35%! My taste palate changed dramatically. As Robbie says, "You eat what you crave, and you crave what you eat."

Through the Recharge and God's grace, I have been healed from diabetes and hypertension and am able to live life for Him to the fullest. My prescription medications have been decreased by 85%! What an investment the Raw Truth Recharge was. I never imagined that this dramatic lifesaving change could take place in twelve weeks. The mountain was too high, the weight too much, the disease too embedded. But God brought it low. With Robbie's guidance on nutrition, an exercise routine, and the choices we make, it is possible. Thank you Father for drawing us to the seminars at Kingdom Bound and bringing Robbie into our lives…our hope was renewed, and we've been restored!

TO GOD BE THE GLORY!

—Bill Nowadly
(Bill has <u>lost</u> 90 lbs so far with The Raw Truth Recharge!)

"For I know the plans I have for you," says the Lord. I did not know how my life would be changed back in August 2014 after attending a three-day seminar at Kingdom Bound given by Robbie. At that time I thought, why not attend the seminars; we have tried every other way to lose weight and have spent money on different products and classes. After listening to Robbie, who is so passionate with her faith in God and her knowledge about healthy living, we decided to join her classes.

We learned a whole new lifestyle, changing our eating habits and exercising. I remember prior to attending Robbie's classes, I had asked the doctor what my goal weight should be, I thought to myself there is no way that's going to happen. After twelve weeks of Robbie's classes I lost more than 35 pounds, my body fat is down more than ten points, I've lost five inches off my waist, and I am down two pants sizes. When my doctor saw me for my yearly visit, they thought the computer was wrong! They were very happy with my health changes and weight loss. I was taken off two medications and my diagnosis of hypertension is gone. I now eat the foods from the earth, which God has given us, read labels to make good choices and exercise regularly. We thank God for bringing Robbie into our lives and teaching us that we do not have to be sick, thick, and tired but can be healthy, lean and energetic. We will continue with our new healthy lifestyle and becoming the people God made us to be with Robbie in our life.

Praise God!

—Laurie Nowadly
(Laurie has lost 50 lbs with The Raw Truth Recharge!)

I've lost 89 lbs making healthy food choices with the Detox and Raw Truth Recharge classes. I've been a marathon runner for 14 years, however I found that I can run and still be fat. Robbie taught me that you can't out exercise a bad diet. I encourage everyone who wants to be healthy, make healthy food choices and increase their energy to come to a Raw Truth Recharge Class or read this book and also do her Raw Cuts program!

—Chuck Roberts

Robbie:

Hi, I saw you on *AM Buffalo*. Whenever I think of health, exercise, etc., you appear in my head. Watching you on the show recently made me realize that losing all that weight on my own was good (twenty years ago) but that I have not been thinking ENOUGH about optimum health, and even though I exercise and have more physical life than an average person, I have not stopped to put all the aspects together. It's not just exercise and losing weight, YOU say, show it and live it. Though I'm an older woman, and physically active, I need to put it all together in a more concentrated, conscious way. Thank you for making me realize that, and for being walking proof of beauty, brains and health. You do know you save lives and plant seeds in hundreds of people you've never met.

I'm not easily impressed, but you have earned my respect for many reasons. I travel in high places and your name always comes up when we are speaking about health and "looking and feeling good." If it doesn't, I make sure it does; rarely need to. You inspire and motivate many. ALL of us inspire the world and each other in one way or another; we just are so busy doing it and it is so much part of us, we don't realize our contribution. I try to remind people we all hold power for the good.

—**Laura Wright**

Dear Robbie: I am so excited to transition into this healthy lifestyle. I have learned so much over the last couple of days and everything makes perfect sense. I want to cleanse myself — mind, body, soul, and spirit. I know I have made the best choice for me to help me with my journey to a healthier me. I have made the choice to put myself first for the first time in my life. Ultimately it will help me to be a better and happier person, a better wife and mother. I know that if I don't do this now, it will be very difficult for me to achieve the many goals I have planned for my family and myself. I want to personally thank you for just being you. You are a role model to me, and you have such a positive attitude that has already rubbed off on me. I came home to my family just spilling everything that I learned. I feel like my life is coming full circle. You motivated me years ago when I was in my twenties, and I always had the commitment to exercise, but what I never truly learned was how to diet the healthy way, how to truly love myself enough to eat the healthiest and best foods for me. I am on a journey and I know with your support, I will be successful. I would always convince myself that organic is too expensive and that I wasn't worth it, but I know now, I am worth it.

I am forty-six years old, and I want to truly live life. I want to live to help my daughter raise my grandson and see my future grandchildren. I want to reduce my depression and anxiety. Everything I have done in the past pushed me further and further away from achieving all the things that are important to me. I have been on a spiritual journey for the last couple of months and I prayed for God to help me to resist eating anything that would not be of nutritional value to me and to help me to find a program that would help me with my journey in life. I am happy to say that He brought me full circle back to a woman that motivated me twenty years ago. There is no coincidence that God led me to Dr. Shatkin, who in turn led me to you. I want to thank both of you for investing this time in me and believing in me. It means the world to me. I truly believe that God brings people into your life for a reason, a season, and a lifetime. I already know the reason He led me to you and I feel that what I am learning from you will be with me for a lifetime.

—Lavenia Dixie

The woman below just eighty-five pounds and transformed her health by following what I teach and preach. She didn't believe when I said that she could change her health, but she needed a wheelchair when I met her. She left my class not only out of the wheelchair but able to push it around the block to get exercise! –Robbie

She said: "My next pic will be at the eighty-five pounds lost mark, and I am getting excited. Then on to reach 100 pounds. Many say older people cannot lose weight, well, God has proven that wrong. I am never hungry and love the food and smoothies. I am learning to cook healthier. No need for the wheelchair to shop or visit doctors. I am not well... yet my life is 1000% better and I am able to do my own housework, take care of myself, and make church every Sunday, often walking to it. I am so glad and thankful for your teachings. NEVER STOP no matter how many like me you meet. God is using you in a mighty way. I love you, Robbie."

—Gaymarie Sparrer

Thank you – thank you – thank you!!!

I just have to share this with you. Getting ready to take my yearly trip to visit my snowbird parents in Florida. In years past I'd be in tears by now trying on summer clothes and bathing suits while packing. Well, nothing fits—BUT it's because everything is WAY TOO BIG!!!!! I am truly so thankful for everything I've learned from you!!! I'm trading in my frumpy skirt-style bathing suit bottoms or something that covers much less!!! Woohoo!!

—Rebecca F.

As I write this on the eve of our daughter's wedding, I am reflecting back one year when she announced her engagement and as God's plan...I met Robbie Raugh.

My husband John and I had decided to make 2013 our year to "go into training" and get in shape for our daughter's wedding. We have always had gym memberships and were all about cardio, cardio, cardio. (However, our bodies did not reflect gym memberships). We never tried to change or paid much attention to what we ate unless we were on a "diet" which never lasted long. As health care professionals, you would think we would not only know better but also do better?

Through Robbie we learned many things: preventing disease is our #1 goal! Another Robbieism: "abs are made in the kitchen." It's all about choices, balancing healthy eating, along with weight training and cardio exercise. Muscle fuels metabolism, by building muscle we both reset and jump-started our metabolism. By making it a lifestyle change and not a "diet," John lost sixty pounds and I lost thirty pounds. We not only feel good, we look good!

After a minor surgery I was unable to exercise for a month. I was miserable. For the first time in my life, I actually missed going to the gym. That's when I realized I had made a transformation! It truly was a lifestyle change for me. For a moment I felt like I didn't know myself! I actually said out loud, "Who are you?" I realized losing the weight for the wedding was just a bonus and our real blessing was we were healthy and preventing disease. The Raugh Truth has truly been a blessing in our lives!

Thank you Robbie, for all you do.

—**Tina Lomeo**

Robbie, you are an amazing person. What a blessing you are in my life! I look forward to growing stronger in my health and faith through this walk we are on together. As I reflect on my past twelve weeks, I would never have been able to believe I could ever lose thirty pounds, get my fat numbers down 12 % and be increasing my weights at the gym to 7.5 pounds. My health has improved significantly and I feel wonderful each day. I can run around my house, and no more rheumatoid arthritis drugs! Amazing!!! You are one of God's greatest blessings to me! Thank you!

—**Jan Plummer**

Robbie,

I couldn't let the night end without telling you how much I have enjoyed the past thirteen weeks (Thanksgiving week was a bonus!). While I felt I was already a healthy eater, I learned that healthy eating wasn't exactly what I thought it was. I forgot that food has flavor, is fun to prepare, and is what we need to nourish the body, mind, and spirit. Since meeting you, I have found myself to be more relaxed, able to focus on the important things in life, and to also tell a story to others who struggle day to day.

As a school administrator, my job is to be an instructional leader and to motivate people who don't necessarily buy into what is best or right. I counsel parents and kids, feed 550 mouths twice daily, wipe noses, and mop floors. And I have to be happy each and every day whether I feel like being happy or not. I would find myself hiding my aches and pains because someone else always had it worse than me. After doing Transitions infused with "Robbie' reality," I have found that it is easy to be happy, to feel good, to not hurt, and to not view some of my tasks as chores. I thank God every day for giving me the opportunity to make a difference in someone's life, for I have a very different perspective these days. You have been both an inspiration and instructional leader of sorts by being my coach, and not just a transitions coach, because it is so much more than that. You have been a teacher, a friend, a comedian, a reality TV star, and chef. I can only thank you for all you have done for me, and for my family, as they have been by my side for the past three months. I am excited to continue with the twelve-month plan...and wish it was a real possibility to work out with you at the BAC (someday I will get there!) Thank you SO MUCH for providing me the opportunity to be a better person for all in my quality world. You are a beautiful person inside and out! It so isn't the weight loss; it's the whole package!" Until our next class, I wish you health, happiness and peace.

—**Maria Chille-Zafuto**

I am so incredibly grateful to God that He has given me the opportunity to do what I love and feel that it matters. There isn't a class or day that goes by where I don't thank God for the opportunities to help others live that abundant life He desires for us.

—**Robbie**

APPENDIX

Helpful Websites

www.robbieraugh.com

www.rawtruthhealth.com

https://procoach.app/robbie-raugh (world wide on-line mobile virtual coaching with Robbie)

www.forksoverknives.com

http://wdcxradio.com

http://www.mydoterra.com/robbieraugh

http://nutrametrixcom/bfit4lifeshop

http://www.essona.com/product.asp?itemid=37&Affid=39 (Powershot greens)

Anti-Cancer Resources

http://hippocratesinst.org
The Leader in the Field of Natural and Alternative Health Care
A nonprofit health institute based in West Palm Beach, Florida, Hippocrates has been the preeminent leader in the field of complementary health care and education for over 60 years. Their philosophy is founded on the belief that a vegan, living, enzyme-rich diet – complemented by exercise, positive thinking and non-invasive therapies – is integral to optimum health.

http://gerson.org/gerpress/the-gerson-therapy/
The Gerson Therapy is a natural treatment that activates the body's extraordinary ability to heal itself through an organic, vegetarian diet, raw juices, coffee enemas and natural supplements.

http://www.oasisofhope.com
Alternative Cancer treatment in San Diego. More than 100,000 patients from 55 Countries have come here and there is a ton of research again focused on diet, exercise, and natural remedies.

http://www.theoriginalessiac.com/renecaissestory.htm
ESSIAC ® is a herbal formula that was used since 1922 by Canadian nurse Rene Caisse in helping people with serious illness, particularly cancer. She had helped thousands of people heal and get their life back.

References

The Holy Bible NIV

Wilson, James L., ND, DC, PhD. *Adrenal Fatigue, The 21st Century Stress Syndrome.* Petaluma, CA: Smart Publications, 2001.

Walker, Danielle. *Against all Grain.* Riverside, NJ: Victory Belt Publishing, 2013.

Walker, Danielle. *Against All Grain Meals Made Simple.* Riverside, NJ: Victory Belt Publishing, 2014.

Meyer, Joyce. *Battlefield of the Mind: Winning the Battle in Your Mind.* Nashville, TN: Faith Words Publishing/Hachette Book Group, 1995.

Fuhrman, Joel, M.D. *Eat to Live: The Amazing Nutrient Rich Program for Fast and Sustained Weight Loss.* New York: Little Brown and Company/Hachette Book Group, 2011.

Blaylock, Russell L., MD. *Excitotoxins: The Taste That Kills.* Albuquerque, NM: Health Press, 1997.

Stone, Gene. *Forks Over Knives: The Plant-Based Way to Nutrition.* New York: The Experiment Publishing, 2011.

Gittleman, Ann Louise, PhD, CNS. *Get The Sugar Out: 501 Simple Ways to Cut Sugar Out of Any Diet.* New York: Three Rivers Press, 1996.

Perlmutter, David, MD. *Grain Brain.* New York: Little Brown, 2013

Healthy Eating for Life for Women by The Physicians Committee for Responsible Medicine. New York: Wiley, 2002.

Rosenthal, Joshua. *Integrative Nutrition: Feed Your Hunger for Health and Happiness.* New York: Institute of Integrative Nutrition, 2007.

Fuhrman, Joel, MD. *Super Immunity; The Essential Nutrition Guide for Boosting Your Body's Defenses to Live Longer, Stronger, and Disease Free.* New York: HarperCollins, 2011.

Hyman, Mark, MD. *The Blood Sugar Solution 10 Day Detox Diet: Activate Your Body's Natural Ability to Burn Fat and Lose Weight Fast.* New York: Little Brown and Company, 2014.

Hyman, Mark, MD. *The Blood Sugar Solution: The UltraHealthy Program for Losing Weight, Preventing Disease, and Feeling Great Now!* New York: Little Brown and Company, 2012.

Campbell, T. Colin, PhD, and Thomas M. Campbell, MD. *The China Study: The Most Comprehensive Study of Nutrition Ever Conducted and the Startling Implications for Diet, Weight Loss and Long-term Health.* Dallas, TX: BenBella Books, 2006.

Warren, Rick, Daniel Amen, MD, and Mark Hyman, MD. *The Daniel Plan.* Grand Rapids, MI: Zondervan, 2013.

Warren, Rick, Daniel Amen, MD, and Mark Hyman, MD. *The Daniel Plan Cookbook, Healthy Living For Life.* Grand Rapids, MI: Zondervan, 2014.

Reno, Tosca. *The Eat-Clean Diet Recharged!: Lasting Fat Loss That's Better than Ever.* New York: Ballantine Books, 2009.

Challem, Jack. *The Food Mood Solution.* New York: John Wiley and Sons, 2007.

Gerson, Charlotte, and Morton Walker, DPM. *The Gerson Therapy: The Proven Nutritional Program For Cancer and Other Illnesses.* New York: Kensington Publishing, 2006.

Miller, Dr. Jennie Brand, Thomas M.S. Wolever, Kaye Foster-Powell, and Dr. Stephen Colagiuri. *The New Glucose Revolution.* New York: Marlowe and Company (Avalon), 2007.

Stepaniak, Joanne. *The Vegan Sourcebook.* New York: Contemporary Publishing, 2000.

Bauman, Edward, MED, PhD and Helayne Waldman, MS, EDD. *The Whole Food Guide for Breast Cancer Survivors, A Nutritional Approach to Preventing Recurrence.* Oakland, CA: New Harbinger Publications, 2012.

Hyman, Mark, MD. *The UltraMind Solution: Fix Your Broken Brain by Healing Your Body First.* New York: Scribner, 2009.

TerKeurst, Lysa. *Made To Crave, Satisfying your Deepest Desire with God, Not Food.* Grand Rapids, MI: Zondervan, 2010.

Balch, James F. and Phyllis A. Balch, CNC. *Prescription for Nutritional Healing: Practical A-Z Reference to Drug-Free Remedies Using Vitamins, Minerals, Herbs & Food Supplements.* New York: Avery, 2000.

Esselstyn, Caldwell B. Jr., MD. *Prevent and Reverse Heart Disease, The Revolutionary, Scientifically Proven, Nutrition Based Cure.* New York: The Penguin Group, 2007.

Turner, Kelly A, PhD. *Radical Remission; Surviving Cancer Against All Odds.* New York: Harper One, 2014.

Moss, Michael. *Salt, Sugar, Fat: How The Food Giants Hooked Us.* New York: Random House, 2013.

Appendix

Covey, Stephen R. *Seven Habits of Highly Effective Families*. New York: St. Martin's Press, 1997.

O'Connell, Jeff. *Sugar Nation: The Hidden Truth Behind The Deadliest Habit and The Simple Way to Beat It*. New York: Hyperion, 2010.

Thomas, Gary. *The Sacred Marriage*. Grand Rapids, MI: Zondervan, 2007.

Sleep Journal Reference: J. Catesby Ware, PhD et al. National Sleep Foundation's sleep time duration recommendations: methodology and results summary. *Sleep Health*, January 2015 DOI: 10.1016/j. sleh.2014.12.010

Vegetarian Sports Nutrition, Food Choices and Eating Plans for Fitness and Performance by D. Enette Larson-Meyer, PhD, RD, Human Kinetics 2007

Davis, William, MD. *Wheat Belly*. Emmaus, PA: Rodale Publishing, 2011.

Omartian, Stormie. *The Power of Praying for Your Adult Children*. Eugene, OR: Harvest House Publishing, 2009.

George, Elizabeth. *A Women After God's Own Heart*. Eugene, OR: Harvest House Publishing, 2006.

Warburg, O. The Prime Cause and Prevention of Cancer, March 7, 2013.

Seyfried, Dr. Thomas. *Cancer as a Metabolic Disease: On the Origin, Management, and Prevention of Cancer*. Hoboken, NJ: John Wiley & Sons, 2012.

Servan-Schreiber, David. *Anticancer: A New Way of Life*. New York: Viking, 2009

WebMD Medical References 2013 – 2014

Follow Robbie on Twitter; Instagram; Facebook; LinkedIn and sign up for her newsletter on her website.

ACKNOWLEDGEMENTS

To my friends in Christ who I have done life with, and who have always been there for me, encouraging me, praying, and cheering me on to follow my dreams, including this book. You are like family to me and I love you all.

To my friends in Christ at WDCX radio who believe in me, supported, and encouraged me, Neil Boron, Keri Cardinale, Brett Larson, Nev Larson. I am grateful to you all.

To the staff, teachers, pastors and friends at the Chapel at Crosspoint in Getzville, NY, for your biblical teaching and continued support for my family and me during life's trials. Particularly Pastor Jerry Gillis, Pastor Wes Aarum, Pastor David Drake, and Leroy Wiggins. I am grateful for you all.

To Linda Pellegrino, Sue Dobmeier, and Frank Pacella, my friends at WKBW-TV's *AM Buffalo*, who have believed in me and allowed me the opportunity to love what I do and feel that it matters. Thank you for all of your support.

To Brenda Alesii and Sandy Beach, my friends at Entercom who have believe in me, encouraged me, and supported me in my career and life. Thank you for all of your support.

To Amy and Joe Bueme, Mike LaManna, Tia Willows, Rick Leugemors, and Norris Tomlinson, for your support and belief in me throughout my fitness career.

To Pastor Matt Gold of Alden Community Church, Pastor Marty Macdonald of Batavia City Church, Pastor John Hasselbeck of Northgate Community Church, and Father Joe Rogliano for all of your prayers, support, and biblical teachings.

To Donna Russo, Wendy Mentor and the staff at Kingdom Bound for your continued support in giving me the opportunity to speak at the amazing conferences.

To my gym friends and staff from Bally, BAC and Catalyst who stood by me throughout the years— thank you for your support and encouragement.

To Ryan Robe, Annette Herrman and the staff at Home Run Creative Services for your continued belief in me, and for your incredible expertise in making the Raw NRG Videos.

To photographers Jim Bush, Sarah Bridgeman, Boryana Georgiev, Raquelle Raugh, and Harry Scull, for capturing some of my life on film.

To Kathryn Radeff, Rebecca Rohan, Christen Morris, Donna and Danielle Silvestri, Valerie Bielmeier, Beth Skorka Zola, John/Kim Wieloszynski, Shanelle Raugh, Raquelle Raugh, Ann Marie Landel, Lynn Briand, Eugene Rijn Saratorio and Jeff Raugh, for your expertise, help, editing, and support on this book.

To attorney David White for your continued support, help, and expertise.

Thank you to The Raw Truth Recipe contributors: Valerie Bielmeier, Beth Skorka Zola, Donna Fournier, Keri Cardinale, Lara Frendjian, Michelle Fisher, and Jeff Raugh.

To my patients, students, classes, and clients, who inspire me with their encouragement to continue to help others because it's making a difference in their lives.

To Joshua Rosenthal and the staff at The School of Integrative Nutrition in New York City for their guidance and inspiration to continue to create the ripple effect to save lives.

I believe in God our Father,
I believe in Christ the Son,
I believe in the Holy Spirit,
Our God is three in one.
I believe in the Resurrection,
That we will rise again,
Lord I believe in the Name of Jesus.
~ This I Believe; Hillsong ~

John 3:16

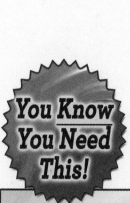
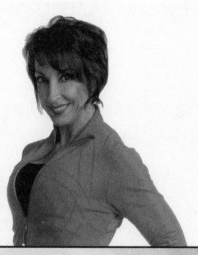
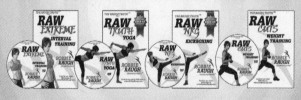
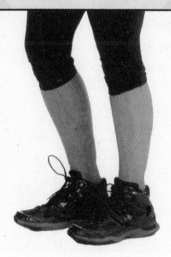

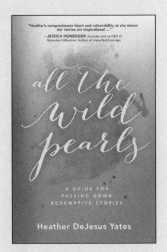
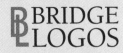

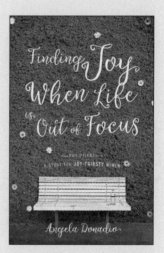
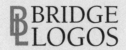

BEAUTY FROM ASHES
Donna Sparks

In a transparent and powerful manner, the author reveals how the Lord took her from the ashes of a life devastated by failed relationships and destructive behavior to bring her into a beautiful and powerful relationship with Him. The author encourages others to allow the Lord to do the same for them.

Donna Sparks is an Assemblies of God evangelist who travels widely to speak at women's conferences and retreats. She lives in Tennessee.

www.story-of-grace.com

www.facebook.com/
  donnasparksministries/

https://www.facebook.com/
  AuthorDonnaSparks/

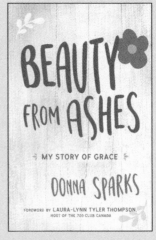

ISBN: 978-1-61036-252-8

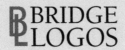

BRIDGE
LOGOS